Sports Medicine for Coaches and Athletes

Older Individuals and Athletes Over 50

Sports Medicine for Coaches and Athletes

A series edited by Adil E. Shamoo, University of Maryland School of Medicine at Baltimore, USA

This series of monographs is devoted to the application of sports medicine research to specific sports. It is intended to present current medical information in a succinct format that is understandable and practical for participants and others directly involved in the individual sports.

This book is part of a series. The publisher will accept continuation orders which may be cancelled at any time and which provide for automatic billing and shipping of each title in the series upon publication. Please write for details.

Sports Medicine for Coaches and Athletes

Older Individuals and Athletes Over 50

Marc A. Rogers, PhD
University of Maryland – College Park

Peter G. Wernicki, MD
Sports Medicine Orthopedist

Adil E. Shamoo, PhD
University of Maryland School of Medicine
Baltimore

harwood academic publishers

Australia • Canada • France • Germany • India •
Japan • Luxembourg • Malaysia • The Netherlands •
Russia • Singapore • Switzerland

Amsteldijk 166
1st Floor
1079 LH Amsterdam
The Netherlands

British Library Cataloguing in Publication Data

Rogers, Marc A.
   Sports medicine for coaches and athletes (ISSN 1024-526X)
   Vol. 3 : Older individuals and athletes over 50
   1. Aged athletes   2. Sports injuries
   I. Title   II. Wernicki, Peter G.   III. Shamoo, Adil E.
   617.1'027

   ISBN   90-5702-600-7

To

Bill and *Lu*
Joanne and *Megan Elise*
Abe, Zach, and *Jessica*

CONTENTS

INTRODUCTION TO THE SERIES

The science of sports medicine and exercise physiology is expanding rapidly. However, this growing body of knowledge is becoming increasingly complex and is not easily accessible to the participants, coaches, athletic trainers, and sports enthusiasts most in need of this material. The *Sports Medicine for Coaches and Athletes* series is designed to explain the scientific basis of athletic performance and exercise training by translating complex scientific data into easily understood, practical information and by providing training, nutritional, and injury prevention and treatment guidelines that are specific for individual and team sports and for various groups of exercise participants.

Adil E. Shamoo, PhD

PREFACE

Much research interest has been focused in the last 10–15 years on various health issues pertaining to the expanding population of older individuals. For example, it wasn't until the early 1980's that exercise training studies were carried out in older sedentary individuals that showed that aerobic training brought about similar improvements in cardiovascular fitness as seen in young individuals and that older endurance athletes who trained the same amount as young athletes had similar performance capacities measured in the laboratory. As far as physical activity and its effect on longevity goes, in 1986 the Harvard Alumni Study reported that those graduates who were more physically active and expended at least 2,000 calories a week in physical and recreational activity lived an average of ~2 years longer than their less active classmates. Since that time much has been learned about how older individuals respond to aerobic and strength training. Furthermore, the safety and benefits of exercise for older individuals and how regular physical activity affects the aging process and the diseases like coronary heart disease, diabetes, obesity, hypertension, and osteoporosis are of continued interest to physicians, exercise physiologists, gerontologists, exercise leaders, coaches and those individuals who run health and physical activity programs for older persons.

We wrote this book because of our strong belief that there are a great number of individuals, including sedentary and active people over the age of 50 plus trained athletes, who would benefit from the information. Because each of us brings his own perspective to the text, this monograph is a unique compilation of ideas and points view. Adil Shamoo has been active in sports, and in addition, teaches sports medicine and serves as a coach, as well. Marc Rogers studies aging and older athletes in an exercise physiology laboratory and is a master athlete while Peter Wernicki sees many older men and women with exercise-related medical conditions in his sports medicine practice. This book is written with both older athletes and older inactive men and women in mind. The presentation ranges from the very simple to the complex, so that older readers without any background in physiology and those with vast knowledge can obtain a well rounded body of knowledge in the area of sports medicine and the scientific aspects of exercise training. It is hoped that more sophisticated readers will delve further into the subject matter via the lists of articles in the "Further Reading" sections at the end of each chapter.

To our knowledge, this is the first monograph of its kind. In all sincerity, we welcome the readers' comments, criticisms, and suggestions for revision. We plan to revise the text whenever feasible. Please write to Adil E. Shamoo, PhD, Department of Biochemistry and Molecular Biology, University of Maryland School of Medicine, 108 N. Greene Street, Baltimore, Maryland 21201-1503, USA.

ABOUT THE AUTHORS

Marc A. Rogers, PhD
Currently an associate professor in the Department of Kinesiology at The University of Maryland and a former National Institutes of Health Post Doctoral Research Fellow in the Applied Physiology Section at the Washington University School of Medicine in St. Louis. Dr. Rogers received his PhD in exercise physiology from The University of Minnesota in 1984. His research over the last 15 years has been in the area of muscle damage, muscle physiology, exercise and aging with over 40 published papers and several review articles in print. A former collegiate baseball and basketball player, he has been a competitive distance runner for 20 years and is a former winner of the St. Louis Marathon. On the "down side" of the aging curve as a masters runner, Dr. Rogers knows about the physiology of aging and activity from a scientific and personal performance standpoint. Dr. Rogers is a Fellow of The American College of Sports Medicine.

Peter G. Wernicki, MD
Dr. Wernicki's educational background includes a BA in biology from the University of Virginia in 1980. He completed his doctorate of medicine studies (MD) at the University of Medicine and Dentistry of New Jersey–Rutgers Medical School in 1984. He served a one year internship in general surgery at Middlesex General Hospital–Rutgers Medical School. Dr. Wernicki then went on to complete a residency in orthopaedic surgery at the Union Memorial Hospital in Baltimore, Maryland. This training included study at Johns Hopkins University Hospital, the Raymond Curtis Hand Center, Children's Hospital of Baltimore and the Maryland Shock Trauma Center. Following his residency, Dr. Wernicki completed 2 fellowships; one in sports medicine and one in arthroscopy.

Dr. Wernicki is currently in private practice in Vero Beach, Florida where he specializes in sports medicine and caring for athletes of all ages. A significant percentage of his patients are over 50 but continue to be active in multiple sports. Dr. Wernicki is a Fellow of the American College of Orthopaedic Surgeons, is board certified in orthopaedic surgery, a member of the American College of Sports Medicine, the Southern Orthopaedic and Medical Associations and numerous other professional bodies.

Dr. Wernicki was a professional and competitive ocean lifeguard for 10 years prior to completion of his medical training. He has stayed active in this field and currently is the medical advisor to the United States Lifesaving Association. He is also chairman of the International Lifesaving Federation Medical Committee. Dr. Wernicki is a competitive marathoner, triathlete and swimmer. He has published, lectured and appeared on television related to numerous aspects of sports medicine. Over the years he has helped treat athletes with the Baltimore Orioles, L.A. Dodgers, Penn State Lions and at the Iron Man Triathlon. He cares for athletes at all levels from pros to recreational, especially in the sports more popular with mature athletes, such as tennis, golf, bowling, etc.

Adil E. Shamoo, PhD
Professor (1979–present) and former chairman (1979–1982) of the Department of Biochemistry and Molecular Biology, University of Maryland School of Medicine in Baltimore. Formerly at the University of Rochester School of Medicine in New York (1973–1979), he also served one year (1972–1973) at the National Institutes of Health. Dr. Shamoo obtained his PhD in biophysics in 1970 from the City University of New York. His research for the past twenty years has been in the area of biochemistry and biophysics of the skeletal and cardiac muscles. More recently, Dr. Shamoo has been studying the effects of dopamine, a brain neurotransmitter. He has contributed to more than 200 research papers. In addition, Dr. Shamoo has edited books and journals, and he has chaired numerous international conferences. He is a member of a large number of professional organizations, as well as having held leadership positions, and is a member of the American College of Sports Medicine. Dr. Shamoo has given more than 200 lectures worldwide on various topics. Dr. Shamoo played soccer and considers himself an older individual who has been active in sports for the past twenty five years as a coach and participant. He has lectured widely on sports medicine. He taught an elective course to medical students on the "Biochemical Basis of Sports Medicine" from 1986–1993.

Chapter

ONE

Basic Physiology and Biochemistry of Aging

With aging there is a general decline in the physiological systems of the body that result in a decrease in the capacity of the heart, respiratory, skeletal muscle, bone, and nervous systems to carry out the physical function that they were designed to do. While these age related declines are difficult to study due to numerous factors, much research interest is currently focused on the problems of the loss of physical function and how it potentially can be prevented or lessened. The presence of disease, nutritional status, changes in body weight, and physical inactivity are all factors that can affect the aging process and so they must be accounted for when trying to define the course of the normal aging process.

Table 1.1. Factors Affecting the Physiological Systems

- Disease
- Nutritional Status
- Changes in Body Weight
- Physical Inactivity

The aging process can best be described as a reduced capacity to regulate cellular processes and organ functions so that there is a decrease in the chance for survival. This loss of physiological control becomes obvious to us by the reduction in work capacity, slowing of reaction time, decreased resistance to illness, difficulty in and the inability to carry out the activities of daily living such as shopping, housework, and gardening that typically occur with aging. The effects of aging on physiological function and human performance are very difficult to measure accurately. Lifestyle habits may alter health status and performance during the passage of time but the aging process is not halted. The factors listed in Table 1.1 all affect the various systems, cardiovascular, respiratory, and skeletal muscle.

CARDIOVASCULAR SYSTEM

The cardiovascular system of humans has an extensive ability to adapt to the demands of regular endurance (aerobic) exercise training. Aerobic training is exercise that uses large volumes of oxygen to produce energy. In exercise physiology, the basic test one uses to determine the capacity of the cardiovascular system is the maximal oxygen consumption test (VO_2 max) typically performed on a motor-driven treadmill or stationary bicycle. The VO_2 max test measures the capacity of the body to take in oxygen, transport the oxygen in the blood to the skeletal muscles where the oxygen is used to produce a chemical called ATP (the energy currency of the cell) that ultimately fuels the contraction of the muscles. In general. VO_2 max is increased between 10–25% after a period of 10–12 weeks of regular, vigorous, aerobic exercise training.

Unfortunately, the capacity of the cardiovascular system and VO_2 max is not maintained throughout the lifetime in sedentary persons or in those individuals who previously were engaged in regular aerobic training that increased their level of cardiovascular fitness. In sedentary individuals, the VO_2 max declines at a rate of 10% per decade commencing at about the age of 25 years. This decline in capacity is brought about by the reduction in maximal heart rate that occurs with aging, along with the decline in pumping capacity of the heart (the cardiac output). The fact that there is a decline in active muscle mass with aging also decreases oxygen consumption in the muscle cells. Other changes in the cardiovascular system include: 1) a decrease in heart volume, 2) a decrease in the elasticity/stretch of the blood vessels, 3) and a decrease in cardiac enzymes that lessen the strength of the heart contractions.

RESPIRATORY SYSTEM

Most living cells in the body utilize oxygen in the metabolic machinery to produce energy in the form of ATP and in the process generate carbon dioxide which needs to be removed by breathing. The respiratory system consists of the lungs with the tiny alveoli, or air sacs, where both oxygen and carbon dioxide are exchanged with the blood in the circulatory system and the airways, the tubes that carry the air down into the lungs. The capacity of the lungs for gas exchange is extensive with a large reserve capacity that isn't really stressed to the "max" unless one is performing very, very intense exercise. The capacity of the lungs begins to deteriorate on a very gradual basis between the ages of about 30 and 60 years in a healthy individual, considerably faster if the person is a cigarette smoker or one who is exposed to various contaminants in the air that they routinely breathe.

The aging effects on the respiratory system are most notable during maximal exercise so that oxygen and carbon dioxide gas transport is not adversely affected at rest or when performing low intensity aerobic or resistive (i.e., weight training) type exercise. Aging reduces the elasticity of the lung tissue and chest wall which contributes to an increased work of breathing. There is also a weakening of the breathing muscles with aging. In conjunction with an enlargement of the air sacs is a decrease in the number of pulmonary capillaries, tiny blood vessels in the lungs where the gases are exchanged. Larger air sacs and few capillaries means that the area for diffusion of gasses in the lung is reduced so that oxygen and carbon dioxide molecules are not as easily transported from the air in the lungs into the blood.

The deterioration of respiratory function with aging parallels the decline in function of the heart so that, unless there is some sort of respiratory disease, the capacity to move air in and out of the lungs (i.e., ventilation) is not significantly affected during exercise in older people.

SKELETAL SYSTEM

Bones/Joints/Muscles

The loss of bone mineral density, also called osteoporosis, is a significant problem in our current society, particularly for older women. Bone density or mass peaks in women at about the age of 30, after which it declines, especially after menopause. Men seem to retain their bone density better than women such that the losses don't become apparent until age 50 or 60 years. The mechanisms for bone loss are not completely understood but the decrease seems to be related to physical inactivity, diet (calcium intake), blood flow to the skeleton, and hormonal factors.

Generally speaking, joints become less stable and less mobile with aging. Collagen fibers (the major protein of connective tissue, cartilage, and bone) are seen to degrade over time and sometimes cross-link with adjacent fibers to increase stiffness. The surfaces of the joints deteriorate with aging and the fluid in the joint spaces that provides for lubrication becomes thicker. Therefore, joint stiffness and loss of flexibility are fairly common in older individuals.

The loss of muscle mass and strength with aging has a direct effect on the quality of life in elderly individuals when they become so weak that it is difficult to carry out household tasks like moving objects, getting out of bed, or rising from a chair. Muscle strength is directly related to the cross-sectional area of the muscle. In other words, the larger the muscle, the stronger the muscle. Muscle strength is relatively well-maintained until about the age of 50 years, after which a decline of about 30–40% is seen until death. The loss in strength is associated with a decrease in the **size** of the muscle fibers and also the **numbers** of fibers decrease. Most studies show that fast twitch (Type II) muscle cells that generate maximum force quickly (as in sprinting and weight lifting activity) are lost to a greater extent with aging than slow twitch (Type I) cells that are more aerobic in character. The loss of fast twitch muscle cells may be in part due to inactivity of these fast muscles in older individuals whose daily activity doesn't require this type of movement pattern. In addition, there appears to be a decline in the number of muscle mitochondria (the power house of the cell where ATP is generated) with aging and a loss of enzymes that help to produce ATP in the various metabolic pathways. So one can easily see that with aging there is a loss of muscle and the ability of the muscle cells to produce energy that enables the older person to do work.

BODY COMPOSITION

Humans generally gain weight as they age, beginning in the mid 20's, up until about the age of 55–60 years, when body weights typically show a decline. The increased body weight is usually the result of a gain in body fat and a loss of muscle, as previously discussed. The average percent body fat in a young male in his early 20's is about 15% while typical for 60 year old men is a percent body fat of about 28%. Young women are usually about 25% body fat and they increase to approximately 39% by the time they attain the age of 60. There also appears to be a change in the distribution of body fat with aging such that older individuals have more fat located internally around the organs, rather than underneath the surface of the skin (subcutaneous fat). This is an important fact to keep in mind since it is the amount of internal fat that is directly related to diseases that we normally associate with the aging process, i.e., heart disease, diabetes, high blood cholesterol levels, and high blood pressure. This is the abdominal fat story where the upper body obesity pattern is likened to the "apple shape" particularly of men. When large and many fat cells are concentrated in this area, fatty acid molecules are available to the liver where they can serve to increase levels of fat and cholesterol in the blood and also to contribute to insulin resistance in the tissues. The lower body obesity pattern ("pear-shaped", if you will) more common to women, while not necessarily being a healthy situation, is much less harmful compared with the upper body distribution. Oftentimes these characteristic fat patterns are difficult to change, but there is hope for people with this problem via programs that combine diet modification and exercise, as will be explained in the last chapter of the book.

NEUROPHYSIOLOGICAL FUNCTION

Assorted neural changes occur with aging and like with the other physiological systems, some of these changes are difficult to sort out from decrements caused by disease or disuse. Changes in neural function include decreased vision, hearing loss, deterioration of short-term memory, decreased reaction time, and a relative inability to process several pieces of information at the same time. It appears that central information processing in the brain is slowed to a greater extent than peripheral responses like movement time and the conduction speed of actual neural signals. There may be a biological basis for the decrease in behavioral speed since it has been shown that central nervous system function slows with aging. Movement speed slows with aging and this can be easily observed as it affects the performance of daily tasks such as driving, walking, handling objects, and so forth. As a safety issue, for example, driving problems and accidents increase with advancing age due to the inability to read road signs, difficulty seeing the instrument panel at night, and sun-glare on the windshield. The end result of the increased accident rates in older persons is that insurance rates are higher, the aged suffer age discrimination in jobs that require the operation of machinery, and job loss in occupations such as an airline pilot or other transportation job where safety of the public is involved. There is some recent information that shows that some of the neurophysiological deterioration with aging may be lessened with regular physical activity.

FURTHER GENERAL READING

Spirduso, W.W. (1995) Physical Dimensions of Aging. Human Kinetics Publishers, Champaign, IL.

DeVries, H.A. and T.J. Housh (1994) Physiology of Exercise: For Physical Education, Athletics and Exercise Science. Brown and Benchmark, 5th Edition, Dubuque, IA, pp. 383-399.

Chapter

I *TWO*

Screening for Health Status Before Physical Activity

Exercise testing and exercise training are generally regarded as very safe for older individuals. In sedentary but healthy men over the age of 40 and women who are older than 50, it is recommended that they have a graded maximal exercise test administered by a physician prior to participating in a regular program of moderate to vigorous exercise training. The Physical Activity Readiness Questionnaire, (PAR-Q), is a simple screening test that can indicate whether or not an individual should be seen by a physician prior to starting an exercise program. Even though exercise tests require that the older individual perform maximal exertion on the motor-driven treadmill or the cycle ergometer, the chances of having a medical problem when the test is supervised by the appropriate medical personnel is very, very small. The results from a

graded maximal exercise test are useful, not only to determine if exercise is safe for the individual, but the data is
also used to write an appropriate exercise prescription
that is tailor made for the older individual. Furthermore,
some of the cardiovascular information gathered from an
exercise test may be used to diagnose an underlying
medical condition of which the person was unaware.

PRE-SCREENING

The screening of potential participants in exercise programs is
important for older individuals for safety reasons and so that
effective exercise prescriptions can be made. Also, some form
of screening should be done prior to having an older person
perform a graded maximal exercise test. This is so for apparently healthy folks as well as for those older people who may
have one of the chronic diseases that we normally associate
with the aging process, i.e., heart disease, high blood pressure,
adult onset diabetes, osteoporosis. The health screening serves
to identify and exclude individuals with medical conditions
that would make it unsafe to exercise. The screening also
would serve to identify people with risk factors and disease
symptoms who should seek medical evaluation from their
doctor before starting an exercise program. Furthermore, the
screening would identify those individuals with significant
disease who should participate in **a medically supervised**
program of exercise.

The Physical Activity Readiness Questionnaire (PAR-Q;
Figure 2.1) has been designed as a baseline series of questions
for subject entry into a low to moderate intensity program of
regular physical activity. This PAR-Q was developed in
Canada to identify the relatively small number of adults and
older individuals for whom physical activity might present a
problem and also for those who should consult a professional
for medical advice about the type of physical activity that
would be appropriate for them.

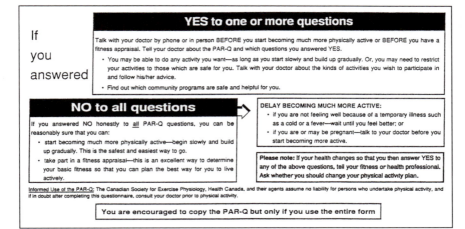

Figure 2.1. Physical Activity Readiness Questionnaire (PAR-Q)*
*From S. Thomas, J. Reading and R. J. Shephard. Revision of the Physical Activity Readiness Questionnaire (PAR-Q) Can J Sport Sci. 17:338–345, 1992. Published with permission.

NEED FOR A MEDICAL EXAMINATION AND CLINICAL EXERCISE TEST

The benefits of physical activity for young and old alike are numerous and will be expanded upon later in one of the chapters of this book. Common misconceptions that exercise is dangerous and that all potential participants who are sedentary **must** have a medical evaluation before exercising contribute to the relatively low numbers of individuals in this country who exercise on a regular basis. It is for this reason that the American College of Sports Medicine (A.C.S.M.), the primary professional organization for sports medicine doctors and exercise physiologists, has put forth very specific criteria for who needs a diagnostic medical examination and/or graded exercise test prior to participation in a program of regular physical activity. A graded exercise test is performed on a cycle ergometer or motor-driven treadmill where the work in speed or grade or resistance is gradually increased every few minutes and the subjects' heart rate, blood pressure, and the electrical activity of the heart (EKG) are measured to make sure that the responses are normal.

In apparently healthy men younger than 40 years and women younger than 50 years, **no** medical examination or clinical exercise test is required prior to participation in a program of moderate physical activity (intensity of 40–60% of maximal capacity) or vigorous physical activity (> 60% of maximal capacity). In healthy older men (40+ years) and women (50+ years), **no** medical exam or exercise test is required for moderate intensity programs of physical activity **but** for programs that are vigorous in nature, a medical exam and exercise test **should** be performed for people in this age group.

For older individuals with 2 or more heart disease risk factors (age, men > 45 years and women > 55 years; family history of heart disease; high blood pressure; diabetes; high cholesterol; smoking; physical inactivity; no activity and sedentary job) and who experience physical symptoms of disease, a medical examination **and** an exercise test should be performed. In sedentary older people who have no obvious symptoms in their daily life related to cardiovascular disease, the performance of a maximal graded exercise test may detect the presence of some underlying disease process.

SAFETY OF EXERCISE FOR OLDER INDIVIDUALS

Clinical exercise testing that is carried out by well-trained and knowledgeable physicians/exercise physiologists/other health personnel is a very safe procedure. Data from over 2,000 clinical exercise testing facilities and 500,000 exercise tests show that with regard to the risk of maximal exercise testing.

- ~ **0.5** deaths occur per **10,000** exercise tests

- the heart attack rate is **3.6** attacks per **10,000** exercise tests

- the risk of a complication requiring hospitalization is ~ **0.1**%

NO CAUSE FOR ALARM AND DON'T BE AFRAID OF THESE STATISTICS

As one can see, the safety of exercise testing is very good since these rates are very, very low (make that incredibly low), much lower in fact than many common medical procedures. The risks of sub-maximal exercise testing on a cycle ergometer or treadmill appear to be even lower than for maximal testing. In sub-maximal testing the subject is not taken to complete fatigue but rather to an exertion level than corresponds to ~ 85% of maximal capacity. In this instance over 130,000 sub maximal tests have been administered and no complications reported so that this form of testing is safe and can be readily performed in various non-medical settings.

RISKS OF PHYSICAL ACTIVITY

Regular physical activity increases the risk of muscle and skeletal (bone) types of injuries and also increases the risk of cardiovascular events such as heart attacks. Even though this fact is true, the number of injuries and heart attacks is very low for healthy adult participants. For instance:

- 1 immediate event occurs per 187,500 hours of exercise
- 1 death occurs per 396,000 hours of jogging in men
- 1 episode of cardiac arrest (heart stops beating) per year for every 18,000 men

THE NUMBERS MEAN THAT EXERCISE IS VERY, VERY SAFE FOR OLDER FOLKS

While the risk of sudden cardiac arrest increases with vigorous exercise in all individuals, the number of episodes is actually lower in men who exercise on a regular basis than in those men who do not exercise or perform regular physical activity. It should be mentioned at this point that there are no studies in women about the incidence of cardiovascular death while exercising. The major cause of death while exercising is coronary artery disease where the blood vessels going to the heart muscle become blocked with fatty deposits. Most of the people who die during vigorous exercise have been shown to have one or more of the heart disease risk factors that were previously mentioned.

In summary then, it has been determined by research studies that exercise testing and participation in exercise programs are safe activities for older individuals, especially those people that are free of disease and are healthy. The benefits of exercise testing and participating in physical activity programs greatly outweigh the small risks involved.

The Bottom Line: Exercise Testing and Exercise Training is
VERY SAFE FOR OLDER FOLKS.

FURTHER GENERAL READING

American College of Sports Medicine (1995) Guidelines for Exercise Testing and Prescription, Williams and Wilkins, Baltimore MD, 5th edition, pp. 49–85.

Skinner, J.S. (1993) Importance of Aging for Exercise Testing and Exercise Prescription. In: Exercise Testing and Exercise Prescription For Special Cases. Lea and Febiger, Philadelphia, 2nd Edition, pp. 75–86.

Thompson, P.D. and M.C. Fahrenbach. Risks of Exercising: Cardiovascular Including Sudden Cardiac Death, In Physical Activity, Fitness and Health, Human Kinetics, C. Bouchard (ed.) 1994, pp. 1019–1028.

Chapter

THREE

Principles of Exercise Prescription

The basics behind exercise prescription for older individuals are quite similar to those for younger people. Begin a strength or aerobic exercise training program at a level that is easily tolerated and then gradually over weeks and months, increase the intensity level of the exercise, the duration of each exercise session, and the number of times that you perform the exercise session per week. This progressive overload of the skeletal muscles and the heart results in positive adaptations that increase the capacity of the cardiovascular system and the muscles to do work. For strength training this generally means 1–3 sets of each exercise with 8–12 repetitions performed at least 2 times per week. For aerobic/endurance exercise training the rule to follow is about 30–60 minutes of aerobic activity at 60–90% of maximal capacity (considered to be moderately hard) between 3 and 5 days per week. For most older individuals a combination program that is maintained over months and years and includes both aerobic and strength training is the most beneficial in terms of overall health status and physical fitness. The ultimate program, of course, is one that is begun and maintained throughout the individual's lifetime.

FOR IMPROVING MUSCLE STRENGTH

Strength training has become a popular activity in recent years both as a means of improving the muscular fitness of athletes, young and old, and as a recreational pursuit for those individuals who are interested in their personal health. It is well known that with aging there is a significant loss of muscle mass in both men and women, as mentioned in Chapter One. This loss of muscle results in a significant reduction in muscle strength. Recent studies indicate that older individuals can increase both their muscle strength and muscle mass in response to a regular program of resistance exercise training. The goal of this section of the chapter is to explain the simple science of resistance exercise training so that the older reader can put together a safe and effective program to either improve muscular strength or prevent its decline with aging. Three Questions are to be answered:

- **What is muscle strength and how is it measured?**

Strength training, also referred to as weight training and more accurately resistance training, is a system where the muscles of the body must move against an opposing force or resistance. This resistance can be in the form of free weights like a barbell, force exerted on some type of machine (Nautilus, Cybex, Universal, Keiser/Air), or other devices such as elastic bands, springs, surgical tubing, etc. Therefore, resistance is the amount of weight lifted or force generated against a machine or device. The simplest definition of muscle strength is the maximal amount of force that can be generated by a specific muscle or group of muscles. Muscle strength is primarily determined by the size of the muscle, the bigger the cross-sectional area of the muscle, the greater the strength of the muscle. For example, a large muscle like the thigh (the quadriceps muscle, in anatomy terms) is stronger than a small muscle of the hand (the pollicis muscle which moves the thumb). At this point in time the reader must become familiar with the concept of repetition, which is the number of lifts performed. Five repetitions is equal to 5 lifts performed throughout the full range of motion. The simplest measure of muscle strength is obtained by administering a 1-repetition maximum weight lifting test (1-RM). A 1-RM is the heaviest weight that can be lifted only **once**. The procedure for the 1-RM test follows:

1-RM TEST

1) Subject becomes familiar with the equipment: practices the movement with the weights or on the particular machine. A warmup should be included where the subject performs several sub maximal lifts or repetitions over several minutes at ~ 50% of maximal effort or in other words, using a weight that corresponds to about 50% of maximal.

2) The subject is allowed up to 5 trials to find the 1-RM with several minutes of rest between attempts; start by selecting a weight/resistance that you guess is just slightly less than your maximal capacity. Increase the resistance gradually to find the 1-RM.

3) The best measures of general upper body strength are 1-RM values for the bench press and military press while the best tests for lower body strength are the leg press and leg extension. Be sure to record the number of trials it takes to ascertain the 1-RM so that the same procedure can be repeated after the training program to measure accurate strength gains.

Another component of muscle fitness is muscular endurance, which is defined as the ability of a muscle or group of muscles to contract repeatedly over time until the onset of fatigue. Common tests are employed to measure muscular endurance such as the 60-second sit-up test for abdominal muscle endurance and push-ups to test for the upper body muscles. Resistance training equipment can also be used to assess muscle endurance by selecting an appropriate level of sub maximal resistance (i.e., weight that is ~ 50–60% of the predetermined 1-RM) and then counting the total number of repetitions that can be performed until fatigue. To measure improvement in muscle endurance after a typical 8–12 week program of resistance exercise training, one would simply repeat the muscle endurance test at the same resistance used in the test before training.

- **How do I plan a reasonable strength training program and how long should I train for?**

THE PLAN

In order to increase the strength of the muscle, its size, or its endurance capacity, a progressive resistance needs to be applied to the muscle, that is, the muscle must be stressed by increasing the load against which the muscle must contract. The muscle can be "overloaded" by either increasing the resistance or increasing the number of repetitions. Usually this overload to the muscle is applied over time, meaning that as one's strength or endurance level increases, the training load is increased as well. In the real world of strength training this means that about every 2 weeks or so, the resistance of the exercise is increased, usually by 3–5 lbs. at a time. When is the best time to increase the resistance? When the weight becomes easy to lift, is the answer. Another way that the training load can be changed is by altering the number of sets of the exercise. A set is a specific number of repetitions.

Muscle strength is best developed by using weights that generate near maximal tension with relatively few repetitions, usually 6–8 repetitions per set. Muscle endurance can be improved by using lighter resistance and 12–15 repetitions. **To elicit improvements in both muscle strength and endurance, most exercise physiologists recommend that older folks use 8–12 repetitions per exercise.** Resistance training for the average, older, healthy, individual should have a flowing rhythm, be performed at a slow to moderate speed and under control, carried out throughout the whole range of motion and not be done while holding one's breath. Resistance exercise, especially with the upper arm muscles, combined with breath-holding can cause excessive increases in blood pressure which can be dangerous for older individuals, especially those who may have even mild high blood pressure to begin with. The take home message here is to breathe normally while performing the exercises.

TRAINING GUIDELINES FOR OLDER ADULTS TO IMPROVE MUSCLE STRENGTH

1) Select a minimum of 8–10 exercises that train the major muscle groups of the upper and lower body. Remember, an important goal of the program should be to improve total body muscular fitness; this should be accomplished with a program that lasts ~ 40–50 minutes.

2) Perform 1 to 3 sets of 8–12 repetitions of each of the selected exercises. At the beginning of the training program start easy with 1 set per workout and then gradually increase the number of sets over the next few weeks as you feel yourself getting stronger. A good guideline to use is one where you feel that you are performing the set to the point of willful fatigue. Then, move on to the next exercise.

3) Perform the training at least **two** days per week. While research has shown that more frequent training and more sets of exercises will increase the strength gains, the additional improvement is fairly small. Recovery is important so have a rest day between the resistance workouts if you are training more than twice per week. Expect some muscle soreness or stiffness after the strength testing and the first few days of training. This is normal and there should be no cause for concern. If the soreness persists until the next training session, this is a sign that one hasn't recovered completely. Therefore take another day off.

4) Perform the exercises throughout the full range of motion at a constant, easy speed with normal breathing.

Table 3.1 Aerobic Types of Exercise

- walking
- hiking
- jogging/running
- swimming
- rowing
- stair climbing
- cycling
- dancing
- skating
- rope skipping
- cross country skiing
- aerobics

5) Exercise with a partner who can assist you and help with motivation.

THE AEROBIC EXERCISE PROGRAM

The important components of an individualized exercise prescription include the mode of activity (or type) which is jogging, running, cycling etc. (See Table 3.1), the intensity, frequency, and duration of exercise plus the progression of activity. The purposes of exercise prescription are to provide for the enhancement of cardiovascular fitness, promote the awareness of health status by assessing risk factors for cardiovascular disease, and ensuring the safety of exercise training. For best results and optimal safety, each exercise session should be preceded by 5–10 minutes of stretching exercises for the major muscle groups and several minutes of warmup activity. Likewise at the end of a session, a 5–10 minute cool down period of low intensity activity and stretching is recommended.

You'll notice that the modes of activity listed in the accompanying table all constitute activities that utilize large muscle groups. This is important for aerobic exercise since it is the large muscles with lots of mitochondria that consume the most oxygen and burn the most calories. Another important point is that these types of activities can be performed for a prolonged period of time and are rhythmical in nature. A wide variety of exercise choices is good for the person who wants to maintain their exercise habit for a long period of time, since skill and enjoyment are fostered by personal choice.

INTENSITY

The intensity of exercise refers to the level of exercise or how intense the exercise "feels" to the participant. The intensity and duration of exercise training determine the number of calories expended. The greater the intensity and/or longer the duration, the more calories are burned. Low to moderate intensity exercise is recommended for most people for several reasons. First of all, low to moderate intensity exercise can be carried out for a long period of time, as previously mentioned, and secondly, the risk of orthopedic injury (like muscle strains, sprains, and stress fractures) is reduced compared with high intensity exercise. What is low to moderate intensity exercise and how is it measured? The American College of Sports Medicine, the largest professional exercise physiology and sports medicine organization of the world, recommends that the intensity of exercise be prescribed at 60 to 90% of maximal heart rate. Maximal heart rate is the highest heart rate that a person can reach when working as hard as possible. It can be measured while walking or running maximally on an outdoor track, on a treadmill, on a bicycle, or it can be estimated, as is most commonly done.

Maximal heart rate = 220–Age (in years)

Ex.: for a 55 year old female: 220 – 55 = 165, that is a maximal heart rate of 165 beats per minute.

To select the appropriate intensity for this individual one would simply multiply the maximal heart rate times the appropriate target range of from 60 to 90%.

Ex.: 165 × 60% (×.60) = 99 beats per minute.

This would be the optimal heart rate to maintain while exercising, which can be monitored by taking the pulse, usually at the wrist, or with one of the commercially available heart rate watches or monitors that sometimes come attached to exercise machines. Usually at the beginning of an exercise program it is a good idea to exercise at a lower intensity, that is, at 60 or 70% of maximal heart rate. As one becomes more experienced and hopefully, more fit, the intensity can be safely increased to a higher level.

Of course, if the simple numbers game just outlined is too hard to follow, there is another way to gauge the intensity of exercise. This method is called perceived exertion or how hard the effort feels to the individual. To use this method one needs to think of the exercise intensity on a scale of 1 to 10 with 1 corresponding to easy effort and 10 being the most intense exertion that one can imagine. For most beginning exercisers then, they should run, cycle, swim, or walk at a level that feels like about a 6 or 7 on the scale. The famous running cardiologist, Dr. George Sheehan, who was also an exercise philosopher and writer suggested to his patients and readers that they exercise at an intensity that allowed them to carry out a conversation with their partner that didn't leave them gasping or out of breath.

DURATION

Time limitations on the part of any individual in our busy world sometime influence the length of time that we perceive we have to exercise. The American College of Sports Medicine suggests that exercise training be carried out for 20–60 minutes in duration, not including the warmup time previously mentioned. Initial goals in the exercise program should be set at about 20–30 minutes per session for the beginning exerciser. If the person is very unfit, then even shorter sessions of about 10 minutes each maybe more comfortable. Some interesting new scientific information suggests that 2–3 sessions of 10 minutes each, interspersed throughout the day may be of benefit for individuals who find it difficult to find a larger block of time. In this situation, brisk walking or stair climbing could be combined with some time spent in the workplace fitness center to total the appropriate dose of exercise for that day.

FREQUENCY

Exercise frequency refers to the number of exercise training sessions performed per week. The American College of Sports Medicine suggests that for those individuals with low to average fitness levels, the ideal frequency is between 3 and 5 times per week. Naturally, the number of sessions performed per week will depend on the individual's caloric/weight loss goals, personal preferences, and time availability with respect to lifestyle. If weight loss is a major focus of the exercise training program, then the objective should be to maximize the total number of calories expended for the week. This means that one should try and exercise probably 5 or 6 days a week, after an initial adaptation period of several weeks when the muscles, tendons, bones, and joints are getting accustomed to the increased physical activity.

PROGRESSION

The final component of the exercise prescription is the rate of progression. This component has to do with how gradually or quickly the participant increases the intensity, frequency, and duration of the individual exercise training session on a week to week basis. For the first 4 to 6 weeks of the exercise program, the intensity, frequency, and duration of the training sessions should be kept on the low end of the range (i.e., 15–20 minutes per session, about 60–70% of maximal heart rate, and 3 times per week). Over the next 4 to 5 months of training, more improvement will be noted if the duration is increased, along with the intensity and the frequency, so that the individual is exercising 3–5 times per week for 45–50 minutes per session at an intensity of ~ 80–85% of maximal heart rate. One can tell if the rate of progression of the exercise program is appropriate if there is not undue fatigue experienced after the sessions the next day and also if there is no evidence of injury. As our running cardiologist, Dr. George Sheehan, used to say, "exercise should leave you refreshed and energized 1–2 hours afterwards, make you more productive and enhance your energy levels throughout the rest of the day." The American College of Sports Medicine recommends that after the initial 6 months of aerobic exercise training, the participant move into a maintenance program where the exercise stimulus in terms of intensity, frequency, and duration can be maintained over a period of months and years. Maintenance and adherence to exercise is vitally important since most people who stop exercising do so within the first 6 months after they start a program. We also know that the old adage, "use it or lose it," is quite true since all of the positive changes in the heart and in muscle function are lost within several months (see later chapter on adaptations) after an individual stops performing regular aerobic exercise training. While "just do it" as a commercial slogan applies to the vast numbers of persons in this country concerning exercise, for the older sedentary person, "just keep doing it" is a better phrase to live by.

MUSCULAR FLEXIBILITY

The exercise term flexibility comes from the word flex, "to bend," and has to do with the range of motion at the various joints of the body. A person with good flexibility in a particular muscle or joint has the capacity to move the body part throughout the full range of motion while the individual with poor flexibility is tight and has a limited range of motion. In older individuals, the flexibility areas of concern are the lower back and posterior thigh regions because a lack of flexibility here is associated with an increased risk for chronic back pain, a condition common to older and unfit individuals. It is well known that chronic low back pain inhibits work productivity and the carrying out of activities of daily living, not to mention the cause of many, many physician visits. Therefore, prudent exercise programs for older folks should include a flexibility component that emphasizes stretching exercises for the upper and lower trunk muscles, neck, and hip regions. The stretching exercises should be performed in a slow, controlled manner with no quick movements.

The American College of Sports Medicine provides for the following stretching guidelines:

◆ Frequency: At least 3 times per week

◆ Intensity: Stretch muscle to a position that elicits a feeling of mild discomfort/tension

◆ Duration: Hold the stretch for 10–30 seconds

◆ Repetitions: 3 to 5 times for each stretch

Individual instruction and guidance from a knowledgeable exercise leader or exercise physiologist is the safest and most effective way to learn the proper stretching techniques for the muscle groups of interest. Remember to emphasize the low back and posterior thigh areas.

● **How much am I likely to improve?**

If one follows an aerobic training program as described previously for about 2–3 months it would be reasonable to expect that your fitness level and exercise capacity would increase by about 20–25% depending on how fit you were to begin with. The less fit individual would improve more than someone who had been training previously.

As far as muscular strength goes, adhering to a strength training program for several months would increase one's strength by about 30–40% depending on how many times per week the individual trained and what muscle groups were tested and trained in the training program.

FURTHER GENERAL READING

American College of Sports Medicine (1995) Guidelines for Exercise Testing and Prescription. Williams and Wilkins, Baltimore, MD, 5th Edition, pp. 153–175; 228–234.

Skinner, J.S. (1993) Importance of Aging for Exercise Testing and Exercise Prescription. In: Exercise Testing and Exercise Prescription For Special Cases. Lea and Febiger, Philadelphia, 2nd Edition, pp. 75–86.

Fleck, S.J. and W.J. Kraemer Designing Resistance Training Programs (Second Edition) Human Kinetics Publishers, Champaign, IL.

Chapter

FOUR

Management of Sports Injuries for Athletes and Those Over Age 50

Sports activities are on the rise in the escalating over 50 population. This has led to coaches and athletes dealing with higher rates of injuries and medical problems. These conditions cover a wide range and can include acute traumatic injuries as well as chronic overuse syndromes. The sites and numbers of these injuries vary somewhat by age and are affected by the normal changes in muscle, bone, and tissue function which occur with maturity. Arthritis and other degenerative processes also become a factor in this age group. A basic knowledge of anatomy plus sports medicine definitions are required to facilitate an understanding of treatment and prevention principles.

The following are some brief definitions that will help with understanding this chapter on sports medicine while some extended definitions can be found in the glossary of terms at the back of the book.

Definitions:

Bone: a lightweight structural scaffolding material that functions to support the body's tissues.

Cartilage: a fibrous type of tissue that lines the joints serving as a shock absorber during movement.

Muscle: a contractile tissue connected to the skeleton that shortens or lengthens thus producing movement.

Tendon: fibrous structures that anchor the muscles to bone.

Ligaments: fibrous structures similar to tendons that attach 2 bones together.

Bursa: fluid-filled sacs located throughout the body where motion occurs that serve to provide lubrication during movement.

Sprains: injury to a ligament that involves stretching or tearing.

Strains: stretching or tearing injuries to the muscle-tendon unit.

Tendinitis: inflammation of a tendon.

Bursitis: inflammation of a bursa.

Immediate treatment of acute injuries centers around the concept of R-I-C-E (Rest, Ice, Compression, and Elevation) along with cessation of the offending activity. Athletes and their coaches need to be aware that an injury which does not resolve quickly on its own may require the services of a physician specifically trained in sports medicine. Eventual resumption of sporting activities needs to occur slowly and carefully under professional guidance. Prevention of sports related injuries centers around an adequate warm-up, appropriate stretching, and a cool-down period. Prevention also entails avoiding excesses which can lead to overuse syndromes. Furthermore, proper equipment, clothing; and footwear are necessary to prevent injuries. Instructions from a qualified coach or trainer may be required to learn the skills and techniques necessary to avoid problems. Finally, as the general population continues to age, more and more older athletes have undergone total joint replacements, thus these athletes need to be aware of the recommended sports and suggested activity modifications that will enable them to continue in a healthy lifestyle.

Between 1990 and 2010, the population over 45 years old in the United States will increase from 82 to 124 million. Numerous studies throughout the years have shown that leading a healthy active lifestyle can improve one's overall longevity and quality of life. This, however, is not without risks, many of which involve injury to the musculo skeletal system. When one generally thinks of an injury, they envision an acute event such as a twisting of an ankle. However, many of the "injuries" that an athlete experiences have a slow and gradual onset. These include overuse injuries, such as tendinitis. Therefore a better term may be athletic-related condition, but for the purposes of this chapter, we still shall refer to all of these processes as "injury."

Due to the inevitable age-related changes that do occur to the body, certain types of injuries are more prominent in the mature athlete, such as arthritic or impingement-related injuries. Overuse injuries appear to be relatively constant between the younger and older athletes up until the age of 65 when they generally decrease. The acute traumatic injuries such as sprains and fractures are, as one would expect, less prominent in the older population. It is unclear as to whether these rates are solely related to anatomic changes. There also may be some effect on these numbers by the relative prevalence of the various types of sports.

ACUTE INJURIES

These are injuries that occur with a sudden onset. In many cases, they are due to trauma, such as a fall while skiing. These injuries may be obvious resulting in fractures, dislocations, or significant ligament damage. The areas involved may be quite tender, swollen, and unable to tolerate movement or weight bearing. However, not all acute injuries are necessarily traumatic in nature. One may be participating in a sport without experiencing any obvious trauma but a body area may suddenly become painful or disrupted. For example, these would include acute tendon ruptures such as the Achilles. This could happen while running or reaching for a shot in tennis.

When an acute injury occurs, the activity should be stopped and treatment initiated. The type of treatment and guidelines on when medical care should be sought will be discussed later.

OVERUSE INJURIES

These are by far the most common types of conditions encountered in sports medicine. Most are due to anatomic areas which become inflamed. They are often referred to as "itis" and include tendinitis, bursitis, etc. They are due to some type of overuse of the affected area. This can be due to doing an activity for too long, for example, running too many miles at one time, or can be caused by doing an activity too hard, such as weightlifting an excessive number of pounds. It can even result from carrying out an activity too frequently such as playing tennis and golf every day when one previously did not play regularly. Other factors can also contribute to overuse injuries, such as poor technique or improper equipment.

Overuse injuries generally develop slowly and are progressive if the activity is continued at its increased level. As a rule of thumb, one should not increase the amount or intensity of an activity greater than 10% per week. A knowledgeable sports medicine professional can help the athlete sort through his or her sports history to deduce the cause of the overuse injury. This includes looking at amount, intensity, technique, equipment, etc. Coaches also need to be aware of these facts when attempting to increase practice or when introducing new techniques. If the causes of the overuse are not found and corrected, despite medical treatment, these conditions will not improve as expected.

ARTHRITIS

The definition of arthritis is inflammation within a joint. There are three basic types of arthritis. By far the most common type is osteoarthritis also known as degenerative joint disease. Degenerative joint disease is a wear and tear phenomena. The cartilage lining the joint wears out over time due to normal or excessive use. Some individuals may be prone to earlier arthritis in various joints due to genetics or biomechanics. The most common areas to develop osteoarthritis are in the weight bearing joints such as the hips, knees, feet, and ankles. Other areas which are prone to develop arthritis include the neck, back, hands, and shoulders. Osteoarthritis develops gradually over a number of years and symptoms can occur gradually or they can occur relatively suddenly with only minimal trauma. The affected joint will be painful to move, to put weight on it, and occasionally to touch. It may also be somewhat swollen, red, and warm. Osteoarthritis is diagnosed by an x-ray and will show narrowing of the joint and irregularity of the bony surface. The treatment includes avoidance of the offending activities along with bracing, oral medications, injections, and possibly surgery. Surgery can be either minor, such as arthroscopy which is used to smooth out the roughened surfaces, or major, such as a total joint replacement in which the actual diseased cartilage and ends of the bone are removed and replaced with metal and plastic components. In general, degenerative joint disease is progressive over time. Strengthening the muscles around affected joints can help delay this progression. Depending on the joints involved, certain suggestions regarding specific sports may be necessary. For example, if one has significant degenerative arthritis within the knees, weight bearing sports such as running would not be recommended.

A second type of arthritis is that of traumatic arthritis. This occurs at any age when a significant injury is sustained to a joint. An example would be a fracture which goes through the end of the bone leaving a displacement within the joint itself. This immediately creates a surface which is irregular. This is, in effect, an "instant" osteoarthritis. The joints involved in this type of arthritis act like and are treated similar to those with degenerative joint disease.

A third type of arthritis is immunological arthritis, the most common of which is rheumatoid arthritis. This is an autoimmune disease which is systemic in nature and somewhat hereditary. Certain cells and chemicals within the body react for unknown reasons against the body's own cartilage and begin to weaken and destroy it. The surfaces of the joints involved are broken down. This leads to excessive swelling and inflammation within the surrounding tissues. Many of these cases of autoimmune arthritis are diagnosed by blood tests and can be treated with medications. Ultimately in severe cases, surgery may be required.

Coaches need to be cognizant of mature athletes with arthritic joints. They should help athletes plan their sporting activities to minimize worsening of their pre-existing arthritis. Those athletes who have had total joint replacements need to discuss sports participation with their physicians in order to prevent future problems.

As of the writing of this monograph, no proven treatment for the prevention of arthritis is available other than routine activity and general conditioning of the muscles around joints. In this regard, athletic individuals should hope to experience less arthritis as opposed to the "couch potato" or inactive person. Numerous studies have been performed which indicate that appropriate, controlled exercise, for example in runners, does not lead to any increase in arthritis within the joints of the lower extremities. Other suggestions for prevention of arthritis include maintenance of ideal body weight. Individuals who are obese or overweight will place increased stress on their joints and therefore have an increased risk of developing arthritis. Certain body alignments or biomechanics may also lead to arthritis such as those who are significantly knock-knee or bow-legged, but little can be done to prevent arthritis due to these alignments.

INITIAL TREATMENT

When an athlete experiences any type of injury including acute or overuse injuries, the hallmark of care involves the eponym **RICE**. This stands for rest, ice, compression, and elevation. This is easily remembered by athletes and coaches and can be applied to virtually any body part in almost any situation.

Rest: This refers to the immediate cessation of the sporting activity involved. A player or athlete needs to stop the game, match, race, etc., and refrain from the using the affected body part. At a minimum, this should be carried out until the area has been determined to have suffered only a minor injury. In most cases, the prudent course is to avoid further use or activity until the discomfort has significantly resolved which may be an hour, a day, or a week. In many instances further injury can occur if an athlete tries to "work through" the pain or if he/she resumes activity prematurely. If the injury involves a weight-bearing area, crutches, etc., may initially be required to further rest the affected body part. In some instances, rest may be facilitated by splints, casts, and braces. Rest, when carried out in relation to overuse injuries, may represent a cutting back in the intensity or amount of the activity rather than a complete cessation.

Ice: Studies have shown that a lowering of the local temperature of a traumatized area will reduce further injury to the tissue, decrease swelling, and provide some pain relief. Ice should be applied as soon as possible after injury and applied on a 20 minute basis at intervals at least several times a day for the first 48 hours. The application of cold can be accomplished through the use of ice in a plastic bag, chemical cold packs, or even the use of a pre-frozen large bag of vegetables such as peas or corn. Ice may be more effective in a wet or semi-liquid state by increasing the surface area to the skin, however, direct contact with the skin should be avoided to prevent "ice burns." After approximately 48–72 hours, ice may be alternated with heat to increase circulation to the affected area and speed healing.

Compression: Application of a light compressive dressing to an injured area such as an ankle, elbow, or wrist can control swelling. It also serves as an adjunct to immobilization in avoiding further injury and reducing pain. The most common method of compression is that of an elastic wrap. Care should always be taken to wrap the body part only lightly to prevent cutting off the circulation.

Elevation: The affected body part when possible should be elevated to a level above the heart. This will prevent additional swelling, decrease further damage, lessen pain, and speed recovery. Elevation can be accomplished by laying the athlete flat or semi-flat and raising the knee, ankle, elbow, or injured area above chest level.

The elements of **RICE** should be started on the athletic field and continued at home until the injury has subsided or until further care is sought.

FURTHER CARE AND RESUMPTION OF ACTIVITIES

It is often difficult to decide which injuries will improve on their own and which require further medical care. Those injuries which are sudden and severe such as a fall from a bicycle with head injury are quite obvious. With significant trauma such as this or in any instance in which there is loss of consciousness, loss of motion of a body part, head or neck injury, or whenever an athlete cannot get up on his/her own, he/she should not be moved and an ambulance immediately summoned by 911. Vital signs should be checked and if the absence of breathing or circulation is noted, qualified persons should begin CPR immediately.

In those injuries in which there is no loss of consciousness or abnormal vital signs, but merely a severe injury to an extremity in which the athlete has severe pain and difficulty with motion of that portion of the body, it is also relatively easy to decide that further immediate medical care is needed. If ambulance transportation is not available or chosen, the injured portion of the body should be splinted or made immobile. This is accomplished by fastening some type of supportive firm object, such as a board to the injured area, thus preventing further movement and damage. Care needs to be taken to assure that the splint is not applied too tight, which could cut off circulation. In any type of extremity injury, circulation, motor activity, and sensation should be checked. Other injuries of moderate severity, such as a sprained ankle, should be evaluated by a sports medicine professional. This is to assure that a fracture or other associated more severe injury is not also present.

The more difficult decisions with regard to further care are in those injuries which do not appear to be serious initially.

The noted principles of **RICE** should be applied. If the injury does not improve over time or worsens, professional care should be sought. Most mild sprains, strains, or contusions should improve in one to two days and most overuse injuries, if mild, should not be worse the day after exercise. If any question exists as to the severity of the injury, it is always better to give more medical care sooner.

If further care is necessary on an emergency basis, the local hospital's emergency room, a nearby walk-in clinic, or your primary care physician should be contacted. For less severe or more chronic injuries which are sports related, a professional familiar with sports medicine should be sought out. In addition, one may wish to seek physicians who are members of sports related societies such as the American College of Sports Medicine and the American Running and Fitness Association. These organizations can be contacted for appropriate referrals to a physician in your area. Often physicians who are familiar with treating athletes will have a different outlook in which they share your goal of returning you to your sport as soon and as safely as possible. They may be able to make more specific and helpful suggestions regarding your injury and suggest causes and solutions including equipment and technique. If further care has been sought with a sports medicine professional, his recommendations regarding return to sporting activity should be followed closely. However, if the injury was minor and did not require professional care, the area of injury should be pain-free or nearly so prior to resumption of any sporting activity. If any swelling or pain with motion is still present, additional time may be needed. The first steps to gradual resumption of activity should consist of gentle motion of the affected joint without weight or stress being applied. Once this can be carried out pain-free, then resolution of normal daily activities such as walking, using the arm, etc., should be resumed. When this is fully pain-free, then light sporting activity can be tried such as jogging or gently swinging of a racquet, club, or other object. Intensity and duration of these sporting activities can then be gradually increased. Ultimately, when one has been able to return to normal athletic form, then competition can be carefully resumed. If at any point along this continuum discomfort or weakness occurs, this indicates that one has progressed too fast and the athlete needs to go back to the last level of pain-free activity and remain there for an additional period of time.

PREVENTION

Not all injuries are preventable, but a large majority of those which we will discuss are entirely avoidable. First, a decrease in the frequency of injury can be accomplished with proper warm-up, stretching, and cool-down periods. Second, intelligent, gradual increase in activity can help avoid overuse conditions. Finally, one must have appropriate equipment, including footwear, for the sport involved and perform the activity with correct technique. By carrying out these suggestions, one will be able to avoid significant injury and continue to enjoy athletics without interruption.

At the beginning of each sports session, the athlete should undertake a brief period of warming up. This usually consists of five to ten minutes of relatively low level lightly aerobic muscular activity. This serves to increase blood flow and temperature within the muscles, tendons, and joints which will increase their flexibility and ability to perform. Such warmup activity could consist of a few minutes of jogging, light hitting of the tennis ball against a back stop, or numerous gentle non-impact swings with a golf club. This activity should not be carried out with any great speed, force, or precision.

Once the warm-up has been completed it is important to carry out stretching prior to any athletic activity. Stretching should last for approximately 10 to 15 minutes. All muscles used during the upcoming sport should be stretched. Specific stretches are available for the neck, shoulders, arms, back, hips, legs, ankles, and feet. Your coach, therapist, or physician can instruct you in safe, appropriate stretches. Stretching should be done in a gentle slow manner in which one applies tension to the musculo-tendinous unit. This is usually accomplished by extending the joint which is crossed by the muscle. This should be done gradually and without any jerking or bouncing movements. Such bouncing movements will actually cause a reflex within the muscle leading it to tighten, not loosen. The stretch should be held for 5 to 10 seconds, then gently released and gradually resumed 5 to 10 times per muscle group. Stretching is best accomplished after the muscles have been warmed up. Special attention should be given to areas of known inflexibility or previous injury. Additional benefit can be obtained by also stretching after the exercise session or sporting activity has been completed.

As mentioned earlier, the number one cause of athletic injuries is overuse. This should always be kept in mind when one considers increasing the duration, intensity, or type of activity they are performing. If one notices any hint of discomfort or problems, keep in mind that "working through the pain" will in most cases only worsen and hasten the problem.

After finishing with your game, match, or exercise activity, it is best to keep moving for a period of time to allow the muscles and other tissues to cool down. This is also beneficial to the heart and lungs which in many cases have been performing at a much higher level than their resting rate. A sudden decrease in their activity level can be dangerous. A gradual decrease will also prevent muscles and tendons from cramping and tightening, thereby further reducing the risk of injury.

Many sports require equipment such as tennis racquets, golf clubs, bicycles, etc. If this equipment is improper due to its condition, type, or size, it may be a cause of injury. Before purchasing any type of equipment, one should consult with someone knowledgeable in its use such as a coach or sales person who can explain the options available. For example, the material, size, stringing, and grip of a tennis racket are all variables which, if not appropriate for the athlete, may lead to injury. Many items become more highly specialized as they become more expensive and directed towards expert or experienced athletes. However, they also become less forgiving and, therefore, the lastest most expensive item may not necessarily be the best for the beginner or intermediate.

While it is beyond the scope of this chapter to discuss each and every sport's equipment individually, one area that can be stressed, however, is that of safety. Protective appliances should always be used when available. For example, mouth guards should be used for any contact sport and protective eye wear should be used for any type of indoor racquet sport. Safety glasses should be worn by any athlete who requires the use of glasses during athletics. Helmets should be used in all sports with a danger of head injury, especially cycling. In males an athletic protective cup should be used in sports in which groin injury is possible. Coaches should not allow their athletes to participate if they are lacking the necessary safety gear. It is also a coach and athlete's responsibility to make sure that the playing area is safe from any hazards and appropriately maintained.

Almost all sports except for aquatic activities require the use of shoes of some type. Inappropriate footwear can lead to numerous athletic injuries. Footwear should be appropriate for the sport. For example, running shoes are made to provide appropriate cushioning and stability for straight ahead running. They do not have significant lateral support for any other type of sport such as tennis, soccer, etc. One should also attempt to obtain a shoe which is best for his or her foot type. For example, many athletes tend to pronate or roll in with their feet. These athletes should obtain shoes which have increased stability and a relatively straight sole. Specific shoe suggestions can be obtained through your coach, physician, or athletic shoe professional. In many cases, orthotics (custom inserts) may be prescribed for specific problems. Finally, shoes, if they are used relatively regularly, only last for approximately six months or four to five hundred miles of running. At that time, although they may still look intact, their cushioning and support has worn down and would subject their wearer to increased injury.

In addition to appropriate equipment, an athlete also needs to perform the sport or activity in an appropriate manner. Improper technique in many cases can lead to injury. An inappropriate tennis or golf swing, a poor running style, or incorrect swimming stroke all can predispose one to injury and problems. When one begins a new sport or attempts to make changes in one's technique, it should be done slowly and carefully with the help of a knowledgeable coach or trainer.

SPECIFIC INJURIES

This section will highlight various injuries which may be experienced by the mature athlete. It would be impossible to discuss each and every injury in detail. However, some of the more common diagnoses will be outlined. Clues to the common causes of these injuries will be mentioned as well as possible treatment outlines. If these injuries are not responding to the general treatment suggestions of **RICE**, then the services of a sports medicine professional should be sought for a complete evaluation and treatment program.

SHOULDER

The shoulder is one of the more frequently injured areas in the older athlete. Problems are common in sports where throwing or overhead motions are used such as tennis, swimming, and weightlifting. Most of the shoulder injuries experienced are from overuse. These conditions can be contributed to by arthritis.

The most common shoulder problem is impingement syndrome. This is a condition where the tendons and muscles of the rotator cuff become irritated and inflamed. The rotator cuff is a group of four muscles and their tendons which overlie and surround the upper portion of the humerus (upper arm bone). They serve as stabilizers for this ball and socket joint and enact certain motions. They can become irritated and painful when they are overworked, especially in activities when the arms are held overhead. This condition can be contributed to by bone spurs which may rub on the rotator cuff. The structure in between the rotator cuff and the acromion (tip of the shoulder blade) is a bursa which can also become inflamed. The older term for this condition is bursitis. Impingement syndrome or shoulder tendinitis/bursitis is felt as a pain or ache within the shoulder which is worsened when the arm is elevated forward or sideways. The pain may be worse at night, after activities, and may radiate into the upper arm. This condition can be caused acutely by a fall onto the shoulder or sudden force applied to the arm. The treatment for impingement syndrome relies on the basics of rest, ice, and anti-inflammatory medication. If problems persist, physical therapy or cortisone shots may be indicated. In some difficult cases, arthroscopic surgery through a viewing scope inserted in several small openings in the skin is helpful for removal of the bone spurs, which allows more room for the rotator cuff muscles. Prevention of this problem is aimed at strengthening the rotator cuff muscles with a series of specific exercises. Athletes who have had or who are at risk for impingement syndrome due to overhead activities should carry out a regular program of these exercises which can be obtained from a qualified physical therapist or trainer. When the impingement syndrome has been present for a significant period of time, eventually the bone spurs can begin to tear into the tendons of the rotator cuff. This is often referred to as a "rotator cuff tear." In some cases this develops gradually without any specific symptoms. In other cases, it may be experienced as a sudden snap or giving way within the arm. If the tear is small, function and motion of the arm may continue to be relatively normal. However, if the tear is large the athlete may have difficulty in raising the arm away from the body. Initially, this weakness could be due to pain or swelling, but if it persists, it warrants referral to a qualified specialist for x-rays and further testing. In older individuals, treatment of a tear may be only for symptomatic relief and addressed at decreasing any pain or inflammation which is present. However, in the athletic population, surgery is usually suggested. Although arthroscopic techniques are available, in most cases an open surgical procedure is required to reattach or repair the torn muscles and tendons of the rotator cuff.

A related disorder of the shoulder is that of a rupture of the long head of the biceps tendon. This injury also occurs in athletes who carry out overhead activities with their arms. In a manner similar to the method by which the rotator cuff is impinged or torn, the bone spurs can wear on the biceps tendon which courses through the shoulder. This tendon can be simply irritated presenting as pain in the front lower part of the shoulder. Conservative treatment is tried first with RICE. If this is not helpful, a specialist may prescribe formal physical therapy with ultrasound treatments or possibly even a cortisone injection. In some instances, the wear on the tendon progresses to the point where it actually tears or ruptures. The athlete will notice that the biceps tendon has sagged and he will find a prominence of the biceps two-thirds of the way down the front of his arm above the elbow. At first this may be somewhat painful and bruised. Luckily, the biceps has a second, shorter tendon, or head, which is attached in a different area of the shoulder. This tendon is not vulnerable to rupture; so, once the initial trauma has subsided, the biceps muscle will function at near normal levels and strength. If a possible tendon rupture occurs, the athlete should rest the arm and be seen by his sports medicine physician for a thorough examination. Surgery is almost never recommended, unless the rupture has occurred at the lower end of the muscle near the elbow. In this case, re-attachment may be required. The occurrence of a biceps rupture, however, often signals other impending problems within the shoulder such as those of a torn or nearly torn rotator cuff.

Another cause of shoulder pain may involve the acromioclavicular joint. This is where the collar bone, or clavicle, attaches to the scapula, or shoulder blade. This joint has only a slight amount of motion and helps to support the shoulder. A fall on or blow to the front or top of the shoulder may injure or sprain this joint. These are also known as shoulder separations. The separations are graded from I to VI with the most common ones being I through III. Grade I is a mild sprain which will get better on its own after several weeks of rest. A grade II sprain requires longer rest and professional evaluation. Due to a partial disruption of the ligaments around this joint, grade II sprains may leave a permanent separation of this joint. This usually does not have any long term functional problems. Grade III is a complete separation of this joint which will result in a noticeable bump on the top of the shoulder. This injury is somewhat painful initially, but the discomfort will resolve with time. In rare instances, surgery may be required. However, research has shown that the functional results with non-operative observational care are equal to those treated with surgery.

Over the years, the acromioclavicular joint can develop arthritis within it which shows up simply as discomfort in the top of the shoulder. This may resolve with rest, ice, and anti-inflammatory medication. If this does not prove helpful, activity modification along with several judicious cortisone shots may further relieve the discomfort.

Even more common than acromioclavicular separations are clavicle fractures. These occurs from a fall onto the shoulder, such as in a bicycle accident. Most clavicular fractures show up as pain, a bump, and grating sensation along the collar bone. Immediate x-rays should be obtained and the shoulder is often immobilized in a figure-of-eight strap or sling for several weeks to allow the fracture to heal. The success of healing in these fractures is close to 100%. Certain distal fractures are, however, more difficult to heal and may require early operative intervention to repair this area of the bone.

While arthritis can develop within the shoulder, it is less likely here than in weight bearing joints such as the knees or hips. Arthritis will usually develop as a gradual ache or discomfort within the arm associated with decreasing motion and stiffness. Anti-inflammatory medication and activity modification are the hallmarks of treatment. X-rays will reveal the extent of the arthritis and your physician can advise you on the level of function and performance you can expect from the shoulder. In more severe cases, an arthroscopic smoothing of the arthritic areas may lead to some additional pain relief. Ultimately in those severe cases where the pain is affecting normal daily activities, a total shoulder replacement can be considered.

The final shoulder condition to be discussed is that of laxity which can have several causes. This condition can occur as a natural state in athletes who have loose connective tissue often referred to being double-jointed. It can occur from over stretching or overworking the joint in athletes who carry out overhead activities such as throwing or swimming. If the surrounding musculature of the shoulder is strong, this may not present a problem. However, if the muscles become weak, the laxity may become symptomatic. Finally, laxity can develop from a traumatic incident such as a fall with the arm outstretched and rotated. Such a fall will often dislocate the humeral head out of the shoulder socket, or it may just partially dislocate. The mildest form of laxity may present itself as a slight instability felt only when carrying out overhead activities such as throwing.

If laxity is felt, the offending activities should be curtailed, anti-inflammatory medications taken, ice applied, and the athlete should seek further care. Physical examination may diagnose the problem or further more specific tests such as a CAT scan or MRI may be needed. Dislocations in those over 30 rarely re-occur without further trauma, however, damage to structures within the shoulder may lead to continued discomfort and laxity. Dislocations in those over 50 may be associated with additional damage such as concurrent tears to the rotator cuff. After an initial orthopaedic evaluation and rest in a sling for several weeks, an aggressive physical therapy program for strengthening of the surrounding shoulder musculature is indicated. In instances where continued pain or slippage is felt to be occurring, surgical evaluation and possible reconstruction to re-tighten the shoulder may be required.

ELBOW

The most common cause of elbow discomfort in athletes of all ages is epicondylitis. This term refers to the inflammation of the epicondyle or bony prominence on the inside (medial) and outside (lateral) sides of the elbow. These are the areas where the tendons of the forearm muscles attach. These muscles are those which flex and extend the wrist and fingers. Pain is the usual symptom and may be associated with weakness of wrist and hand activities.

Lateral epicondylitis, or that located on the outside of the elbow, is often referred to as tennis elbow, although in most cases, it is not brought about by tennis. It can occur from any type of gripping activity including golf, softball, bowling, weight-lifting, or even cycling. Often, it is related to occupational activities such as typing or computer use or even such leisure activities as knitting or crocheting. Medial epicondylitis, or that occurring on the inside of the elbow, can occur with any of the above activities and is seen even more commonly with golf. Medial symptoms are more recalcitrant to treatment and may involve some irritation of the nearby ulnar nerve giving a feeling of numbness or "pins and needles" in the hand.

Epicondylitis can be seen in those athletes who are increasing or changing their activity levels. It can be due to learning a new technique, such as a spin being put on a tennis serve. It may even be related to one's equipment, such as a racquet handle that is too large or too small. Another common way to experience this condition is as in the golfer who has taken an errant swing and struck the ground resulting in a large divot. Initial treatment of epicondylitis consists of RICE. The offending activity should be avoided or at least scaled back and equipment and technique should be checked. Anti-inflammatory medication like advil or ibuprofen may be helpful. A tennis elbow band is a beneficial treatment aid and consists of a velcro strap which is applied to the forearm just below the area of discomfort usually with an air or gel pad. This is worn by the athlete for sporting and other activities involving the arm. The brace serves to alter the biomechanical pull, thereby reducing the strains applied and allowing the area to heal. In many mild cases, the condition will improve with these conservative suggestions. If the pain continues, sports medicine physicians may prescribe formal physical therapy including ultrasound and other types of bracing. Consideration may also be given for a localized cortisone injection to further decrease the inflammation. Once the initial inflammation and discomfort has improved, an exercise regimen consisting of specific forearm stretches and strengthening exercises will allow for further improvement, enable resumption of sports, and ultimately prevent recurrences. Other areas of tendinitis about the elbow include inflammation or irritation of the triceps tendon where it joins the tip of the elbow, or tendinitis of the biceps where it joins the proximal forearm. If these areas become painful after or during activities, rest, anti-inflammatory medication, ice, and gradual resumption of activities usually suffice. Arthritis can occur within the elbow and although it is usually not problematic it shows up as stiffness and aching pain after activity. Bone spurs can develop about the elbow preventing full range of motion. The pain may be controlled with activity modification and anti-inflammatory medication. If stiffness and decreased motion is the major problem, certain arthroscopic or other surgical procedures may be beneficial in gaining further motion. X-rays and evaluation by a sports medicine specialist should be obtained.

Another common elbow condition that occurs is olecranon bursitis. There is a moderate size bursa located over the tip of the posterior elbow. If this area is irritated either by a blow or constant pressure, the bursa may become inflamed and fluid filled. This is usually pain-free and does not present any limitations. It can be unsightly and range from a small minimally noticeable bump to a large golf ball size swelling. Treatment initially consists mainly of avoiding any type of pressure or re-injury to the area. Elbow pads can be purchased to apply a light pressure and protection to this region. Anti-inflammatory medications and ice may help decrease the swelling. If the bump is large or not improving your physician may choose to drain the fluid, and in rare cases where it continues to recur, surgical excision may be suggested.

Irritation to the ulnar nerve was previously discussed in relation to epicondylitis. This can also occur without any surrounding tendinitis. The causes may be a direct blow to the inside of the elbow or overuse from repetitive motions. The ulnar nerve which travels down the inside of the arm can become inflamed and begin slipping in and out of its groove. In addition to the localized medial elbow pain, there is often pain that goes down the forearm and numbness within the small and ring fingers. Treatment for this condition includes rest, ice, and anti-inflammatory medication. Bracing may be required to decrease the irritation to the nerve. If discomfort persists, or if the numbness and symptoms within the hand become significantly severe, electronic testing and surgical release of the nerve may be required.

Athletes may experience trauma to the elbow through falls or direct blows. If acute injuries occur and are associated with pain and swelling or decreased motion which does not quickly get better, evaluation including x-rays should be sought. Various types of fractures can occur about the elbow, some which may require surgery to allow for return to normal motion and strength.

WRIST AND HAND INJURIES

The wrist and hand can be injured in numerous ways with almost any type of athletic activity. Injured fingers need to be checked to assure that there is still normal alignment, motion, sensation, and circulation.

The nails and tips of the fingers are quite vulnerable to crushing and may result in a fracture. Crush injuries usually warrant medical care and x-rays. Injury to the nail may result in future growth irregularities within the nail itself. One may experience a hematoma (or bruise) which is a collection of blood underneath the nail. This can be extremely painful and disruptive to the nail. When this occurs, the pressure needs to be released by heating and sterilizing a paperclip, and then using the tip to gently puncture a hole in the top of the nail. Resolution of injuries to the nail bed may ultimately take several months.

Any type of laceration to the hand or fingers can be quite serious and may involve damage to the nerves, blood vessels, ligaments, or tendons which are quite complex and often require surgical repair. Any type of deep or questionable laceration should be evaluated by a professional to assess the need for sutures or further repair. Initial first aid involves applying pressure to the injured area to stop bleeding. This should be followed by elevation of the extremity and splinting the finger with some type of straight firm object such as a popsicle stick, pen, or short board. A serious concern with open hand injuries is the possible development of infection which can occur even through small cuts or abrasions. If one notices any significant swelling, redness, drainage, increased pain, further evaluation is mandatory.

The hand and digits may be subject to numerous sprains or fractures. These may be obvious with notable deformity requiring realignment by a physician. At other times, they are more subtle and may initially appear simply as a "jammed finger," which often occurs in basketball and similar sports. An injury which presents simply as a swollen, painful and mildly stiff joint after an acute trauma should not be taken lightly. These require an x-ray to assure that there is no subtle fracture or significant sprain. Treatment can include splinting, limited use, and possibly physical therapy for a period of time. The fingers can also become dislocated and should be reduced only by a professional, followed by a prescribed period of splinting and therapy. One common area of significant ligament damage is at the base of the thumb. The most frequent injury seen in skiers is a tear in the ulnar collateral ligament of the thumb which is located at the base of the crease between the thumb and index finger. This is usually caused by a fall on the hand as it grips a ski pole. Pain at this joint and instability may be noted when this area is injured. Rest, ice, and splinting are initially recommended, followed by medical evaluation. Surgery is often required to repair this torn ligament. This condition is also referred to as a gamekeeper's thumb.

A fall or twisting injury to the wrist may result in a simple sprain which presents as mild localized discomfort. Limiting one's activities, applying the principles of **RICE**, and possibly wearing a short brace for several days should result in improvement. If this does not occur quickly, an examination by an orthopaedic specialist should be sought. It is difficult to tell the difference between a significant sprain or a relatively small fracture without x-rays. Fractures to this area may be treated with a cast or occasionally with surgery to restore normal alignment. Wrist fractures are common in roller blading and for this reason wrist guards and other protective gear should always be worn.

Various non-traumatic conditions can develop within the hand from sports activities. These problems are usually due to overuse activities either through repetitive grasping or pressure from bicycle handlebars, bats, racquet, weights, etc. Non-traumatic wrist injuries fall into two major categories: tendinitis and nerve irritations. Tendinitis can be seen in either the flexor — palm side tendons or the extensor — back of the hand tendons. These may become sore and swollen, and painful to move. One particularly common area to develop this tendinitis is on the top and base of the thumb extending up the forearm. This is called de Quervain's tendinitis and results from swelling of the thumb extensor muscles as they pass through a small tunnel at the base of the finger. The pain is usually increased as the thumb is forcibly flexed. **RICE** should be tried initially, but formal therapy and splinting may be required. For more difficult cases, injections and possibly even surgery to release and enlarge this tunnel are helpful.

Nerve problems within the hand include such problems as bowler's thumb, in which the side of the thumb becomes painful from direct pressure as the ball is released, leading to localized irritation and hypersensitivity. Splints, technique modification, rest, and medications can be used to resolve this problem. Bicyclists often develop irritation to the ulnar nerve which supplies sensation to the small and ring fingers. This is due to direct pressure on the palm of the hand as one cycles. Numbness and pain within these fingers which does not resolve shortly after the activity has ceased should be investigated. The use of padded handlebars or gloves and changing positions to include different areas of the handlebars or aerobars may be helpful in the prevention of this condition.

Any type of activity, especially sports which involve repetitive use of the hand, can lead to inflammation within the carpal tunnel. This is an area within the wrist through which passes multiple tendons and the median nerve. This nerve supplies sensation and some motion to the thumb, index, and middle fingers. When this area is irritated, one may experience pain, burning, and numbness within these fingers. It is often worse with activities and at night. Initial symptoms should be treated with rest, anti-inflammatory medications, and the use of a small wrist brace. If the symptoms continue or if the numbness and pain is more than intermittent, additional treatment and possibly even surgical release is sometimes required.

An additional condition that may develop within the hands is that of a trigger finger. This can develop from activities which require repetitive or strenuous gripping such as racquet sports. Initially one will experience a snapping or catching sensation on flexing and extending any one of the fingers. There may be discomfort on the palm side of the finger involved caused by swelling of the tendon. Treatment consists of the usual steps, avoidance of the offending activity, anti-inflammatory medications, and ice. One's physician may prescribe physical therapy, splinting and possibly a cortisone injection to decrease the inflammation. If this is not helpful, a small surgical procedure to release the area of constriction will cure the injury.

NECK

Conditions that athletes experience within the neck and upper back can be divided into two categories: those due to acute trauma and those which are experienced over time. An acute neck injury should be considered with any trauma where the neck is forcibly hyper flexed or extended. Any serious head injury may also involve a neck injury. Severe injuries can be accompanied by paralysis of the extremities or even loss of the ability to breathe on one's own. Serious neck injuries include fractures, dislocations, herniated discs, or a combination of any of these. Any trauma to the head and neck needs to be treated as if there is a serious injury present. Help should be summoned immediately. The ABCs of resuscitation should be carried out and the person's neck and back should immediately be kept from any further movement. If the patient is on the ground, they should be kept there until help arrives. If an initial injury is present, further movement may cause damage to the spinal cord resulting in paralysis and significant worsening of the initial condition. Once professional rescue personnel arrive, they will take steps to stabilize the patient and further immobilize the neck and back for transport to a hospital.

Lesser injuries such as moderate aches, pains, and muscle spasms can be due to overuse. This can occur when repetitive motions of the neck, especially in a twisting manner, are performed in practicing various sports. Neck pain can even be caused by generalized muscle tension and stress from intense concentration during sports. Discomfort and spasm from these non-traumatic injuries are due to the muscles surrounding the neck becoming irritated or inflamed. The underlying presence of associated problems such as arthritis can predispose one to problems. In the large majority of these cases, non-traumatic neck pain is not serious and will respond to conservative treatment. Initial care as always involves rest, ice, anti-inflammatory medication, and decreasing neck motion. A soft cervical collar may be helpful, especially for wear at night for several days. After approximately 24 hours one should switch from ice to heat to help decrease muscle spasm. If neck discomfort does not subside, professional sports medicine care should be sought. The athlete's physician may carry out x-rays or further tests and may prescribe muscle relaxants, physical therapy, and/or exercises.

If at any time the athlete experiences dizziness, lightheadedness, radiation of the discomfort into the arms or legs, numbness or weakness in the extremities, or any change in bowel or bladder habits, immediate care should be sought. These symptoms may be clues to more serious underlying problems, such as a herniated disc. Disc herniation occurs when the soft tissue material of the disc that is present in between the vertebral bodies of the cervical spine moves from its normal position and presses on the spinal cord or its nerves. If not treated appropriately, these symptoms may not improve and actually may progress to more permanent damage.

A related nerve injury can be seen in contact sports where the neck is over flexed to either side. This motion stretches the nerves which have just exited from the spine. The athlete will experience a sensation in which he or she loses all feeling and use of his arm for a period of seconds. It then can quickly improve and return to normal in a matter of minutes. This is called a "burner" and its occurrence may or may not be serious. If one experiences this type of injury, they should cease their activity, rest the extremity, apply ice, and be seen by a physician within the next several days.

LOWER BACK

Lower back injuries in many ways are similar to those of the neck. Again they can be divided into two classes: acute injuries that may involve a fall or other strenuous force applied to the lower back, and those lesser more chronic overuse injuries. Any acute injury which results in sudden significant pain within the back should be treated as serious. The athlete should not be moved until rescue personnel can immobilize the individual for transport, x-rays, and evaluation. Those athletes who have pre-existing osteoporosis or loss of calcium from their bones, especially women, are at increased risk of compression fractures to the vertebral bodies of the lumbar spine. These fractures can be extremely painful and may result from relatively minor falls or trauma.

Herniated discs are more common in the lumbar or lower spine and these result in significant pain with radiation down one or both legs. Disc herniations may or may not be associated with weakness, numbness, and bowel or bladder problems. The presence of any of these symptoms warrants immediate attention by a trained physician.

As with the cervical spine, most conditions show up within the lower back resulting from athletics are merely sprains and strains due to overuse. Generalized ache within the lower back associated with spasm are the hallmarks of a low back strain. Cessation of the offending activity, rest in a relatively recumbent position, i.e., in bed for a short period of time, application of ice for 24 hours and then heat, as well as anti-inflammatory medication, usually lead to improvement within one to two days. If improvement does not occur, an exam by a sports medicine physician should be sought. Again, underlying arthritis may pre-dispose one to back problems. If one has a history of lower back problems or arthritis, activities which involve strain on the lower back through twisting or bending should be avoided. Most athletes can help prevent lower back problems if they carry out a regular lower back stretching and strengthening program. Even a history of chronic back problems can be relieved or eliminated with a proper exercise regime.

One final low back condition which deserves mentioning is that of spinal stenosis. As we age, arthritis can develop around the joints of the lower back. This leads to a narrowing or stenosis of the spinal canal and the openings in which the nerves exit the spine en route to the lower extremities. When this stenosis becomes moderately severe, increased activity of the back leads to swelling in this region and increased pressure on the nerves. This compression results in symptoms of pain within the thighs or calves. This pain is often relieved by stopping the activity whether it be sports or merely walking. Occasionally, bending leads to improvement, and after several minutes the discomfort is resolved. A similar type pain to that of stenosis may be caused by vascular insufficiency. In this condition, the arteries supplying the lower extremities have narrowed due to atherosclerosis. Increased muscle use in the legs leads to a relative ischemia (the cardiologist's term for "lack of blood flow") of these muscle groups. This ischemia is experienced as pain and mild weakness. Cessation of the activity will usually lead to resolution of the pain. Patients with this condition find that they can walk for only a certain distance, such as several blocks, before the symptoms develop. They then need to rest until the pain stops and can then continue to walk. If one experiences this type of activity induced pain or discomfort within the legs, a visit to one's physician is warranted. Treatment may consist of activity modification, medications, or in many cases surgery.

HIP

Various conditions can show up as pain in the hip. One common misconception involves discomfort which is present within the buttocks or posterior hip region which radiates somewhat down into the thigh. In many cases, this "hip pain" is not due to any hip pathology, but is actually due to radiating pain from a lower back disorder and should be treated as such. Discomfort felt on the outside hip region may be due to hip bursitis. This type of pain can be pinpointed by palpation (feeling with the sense of touch). It is usually present over the bony prominence of the upper femur. Bursitis may occur due to trauma to this area such as from a fall. In most cases, however, bursitis is related to overuse from the repetitive rubbing of the overlying tendon. Runners, cyclists, swimmers, and other athletes involved in repetitive leg motion may be susceptible to developing this bursitis. The pain may radiate minimally down the lateral leg. Initial treatment involves the basics of **RICE**. Hip bursitis can be further treated and possibly prevented by stretching exercises for the lateral hip structures. If the condition persists, your physician may prescribe formal physical therapy or cortisone injections to relieve the problem.

Hip pain which is experienced in the front of the hip or groin region may be due to arthritis or degenerative changes present within the hip. This is to be considered if the symptoms are associated with stiffness. The discomfort is usually worse after an activity and weight bearing. Rest and anti-inflammatory medications may be helpful. Your physician will x-ray your hip to confirm the diagnosis and recommend further treatment, possibly even a hip replacement.

Another condition which may cause a similar type of groin or anterior hip pain is that of a stress fracture. This can occur within the femoral neck just below the ball of the hip joint. This is an overuse injury occurring in sports involving repetitive weight bearing to the leg, such as running. If hip pain in this region occurs and is unrelieved by brief rest, x-rays or further studies including a bone scan may be needed to rule out this conditon.

Finally, groin pain may also represent a hernia which is an "out pouching" or protrusion of the abdominal contents. Hernias may or may not be uncomfortable. They may occur without significant trauma or they may occur after a stressful movement such as weightlifting. If an athlete experiences a swelling in the groin or anterior abdomen, his or her physician should be seen for further evaluation. Luckily, the most common hip/thigh injuries are simply muscle strains. The type of muscle strain present depends on the area of discomfort. Those within the front of the thigh are quadriceps strains, those within the inner thigh are adductor strains, and those present within the posterior part of the thigh are hamstring strains. Strains can develop during any stressful lower extremity sporting activity including running, tennis, basketball, swimming, etc. Severe strains may actually represent torn muscles or tendons and these can be associated with significant pain, swelling, and bruising of the region. The athlete would notice the onset of these conditions by pain, inability to continue exercising, and possibly even a limp. Severe muscle strains may take several weeks to months to resolve. Initial treatment involves all of the **RICE** modalities, especially ice. An examination by a physician who may prescribe early physical therapy for faster return to activity is recommended. Ultimately, significant stretching activity is required to prevent recurrence of these strains.

KNEE

The knee is the **most commonly injured joint** in sports. Injuries can be either traumatic, non-traumatic overuse injuries, or a combination of both. When an acute knee problem occurs, one should cease the activities that they are performing. If the initial pain is severe and associated with significant swelling and decreased knee motion, one should limit weight bearing on the leg and seek medical evaluation. If you suspect a fracture, the knee should be splinted to prevent further movement and injury. Fractures may require surgery and/or casting. Dislocations of the knee joint are quite rare and are usually only associated with severe trauma, such as a motor vehicle accident. However, the one dislocation which can occur commonly about the knee is that of a patellar dislocation, which will be discussed below.

In those injuries which do not appear to be initially serious, one should stop the sports activities they are performing and apply the methods of **RICE**. The leg should be elevated, compression applied with an Ace bandage or a brace, and ice applied. If the knee improves over the next several hours to days and does not appear to be limiting ambulation, motion, or activities, then one can gradually resume sports as tolerated. If the pain or other problems such as swelling and instability continue for longer than several days, formal treatment should be sought. Your physician may recommend an MRI to evaluate the ligaments, cartilage, and other soft tissue structures within the knee.

LIGAMENT INJURIES

The knee is supported by four main ligaments. The medial collateral ligament supports the inner side of the knee. Injuries to this ligament occur when the knee sustains a force during a sporting activity in which the foot or distal part of the leg is forced away from the body. This creates a strain on the inner structures of the knee. One correspondingly feels discomfort in this medial area which is worse with motion and activities. Depending on the severity of the sprain, this discomfort may be mild or severe. This is usually a sudden type injury and the player will have to stop the activity involved. If the methods of **RICE** do not relieve the discomfort within a day or so, then care should be sought. Medial collateral ligament injuries are in most cases treated conservatively with bracing, rest, physical therapy, and anti-inflammatory medication. It may, however, take several weeks before pain-free activities may be resumed.

The lateral collateral ligament is the reciprocal structure to that of the medial collateral ligament. It provides stabilization to the outside of the knee. It is injured when a force or strain is applied to the knee in which the foot is forced inward. The discomfort is now present laterally and may be associated with swelling, redness, and pain with motion or weight bearing depending on the severity of the injury. Treatment is similar to medial collateral injuries as described above.

The anterior cruciate ligament is the ligament which is located in the center of the knee. It prevents excessive forward displacement at the tibia (lower leg bone) on the femur (upper leg bone). It is often injured by a blow to the knee or in an injury where the leg is planted and quickly twisted. This injury can result in significant pain and swelling, although sometimes it is surprisingly benign in its initial appearance. Afterwards, the knee can be unstable and the athlete may experience a "giving away". As with other possible ligament injuries, one should cease participation in the sport, carry out **RICE**, and seek further evaluation when continued pain or discomfort is felt with activity. The diagnosis is made on physical examination indicating increased laxity or with an MRI. In younger patients who are quite active in sports, an anterior cruciate ligament reconstruction may be entertained. However, in older or more mature athletes, surgery is usually not required except for the treatment of other associated injuries such as meniscus tears. In the mature athlete, the standard care consists of initial rest and conservative measures followed by an aggressive rehabilitation program to strengthen the surrounding musculature. If one wishes to continue in sports requiring twisting or cutting activities, a custom de-rotation brace is suggested.

MENISCUS INJURIES

In between the tibia and femur of the knee are the two cartilage structures of the medial and lateral meniscus. These cres-
cent shaped fibrous cartilages act to provide support and
cushioning within the knee. They can be torn by twisting
injuries or they may be injured from chronic degeneration.
Meniscus tears show up as either moderate acute injuries or
as a chronic discomfort within the knee with an unknown
cause. The knee may experience intermittent swelling and/or
a locking sensation. There will be pain along the inner or
outer side of the knee which is worse after activity, especially
with any twisting motion. In athletes who are beyond the ado-
lescent years, most tears within a meniscus will not heal and,
therefore, not improve with conservative treatment. If one
believes that they are experiencing a meniscus tear, they
should try the initial methods of **RICE**. If not improved, they
should seek care of a physician who may recommend an MRI
or arthroscopy to further diagnose the problem. With arthroscopic micro surgery, the surgeon can diagnose and evaluate
the tear. If it is a peripheral tear, a repair with sutures may be
entertained. In most cases, however, trimming or smoothing
of the area around the tear is carried out. Usually, this results
in relief of pain and allows the athlete to return to his or her
former level of activity. Arthroscopy is an outpatient surgical
procedure in which a small fiberoptic instrument is inserted
within the knee to evaluate the problem. Micro instruments
are then used to repair the tissues. Afterwards the patient
usually can bear weight as tolerated and may require physical
therapy with resultant return to normal activities after several
weeks.

EXTENSOR MECHANISM PROBLEMS

The extensor mechanism of the knee includes the quadriceps
(quads) muscles which are the anterior part of the thigh that
extends the lower leg when sitting. The quads are connected
to the patella by the quadriceps tendon. The patella is the
kneecap which acts as a fulcrum of the knee. Finally, the
extensor mechanism includes the patellar tendon which links

the patella to the upper tibia. Injuries to this mechanism can be acute with a traumatic injury resulting in a rupture in the tendons or a fracture of the patella. Any of these injuries are severe and result in marked bruising, swelling, and pain. The patient will be unable to stand or straighten the knee. These injuries should be treated with splinting and immediate evaluation. Extensor ruptures often require surgical repair and cast immobilization for several months followed by extensive physical therapy but with the appropriate treatment, the senior athlete or exerciser can return to normal activities.

Another type of extensor injury is that of a patella dislocation. The patella normally glides centered within the groove of the distal femur. In some patients, this groove is rather shallow, or the patient's musculature is lacking. This tends to cause the patella to track in a lateral or outside position. If the patient sustains a sudden load to the knee or twisting injury, the kneecap may slip out of the groove to the outside of the knee. This is known as a patella dislocation and is significantly painful. Often with straightening of the knee, the patella spontaneously relocates. In other instances, relocation by manipulation in the emergency room is required.

Treatment of a patellar dislocation consists of immobilization in either a cast or a brace with the knee in extension for several weeks, followed by physical therapy and bracing. In rare instances, if the patient experiences multiple dislocations with little or no trauma, surgery may be required to realign the patella. If one has not experienced patellar dislocation before they enter their 40s or 50s, it is relatively unusual to have it occur in the mature athlete. If the patella only partially dislocates, this is known as subluxation. In a routine subluxation without additional problems, treatment usually relies on rest, bracing, ice, and aggressive muscular strengthening to prevent future subluxations.

The extensor mechanism may also be problematic in nontraumatic injuries. Patello-femoral syndrome is a condition in which the back of the patella is irritated or roughened due to irregular pressure. This can occur from muscle imbalance in which the patella is tracking within the groove either laterally or in a tilted manner. This can be exacerbated by overuse. Usually offending activities involve bent knee motions such as using a stair climber, cycling, running on hills, or working out with exercise machines. Trauma can play a role when the kneecap is struck anteriorly, thus driving it into the femur and bruising the posterior surface. The athlete can experience anterior pain or catching within the knee when bent and he or she may even describe this as a giving way or mild instability feeling. Patellofemoral syndrome is also known as chondromalacia and is more common in women. If an athlete believes he or she is experiencing a patellofemoral inflammation, the offending activity should be reduced in frequency or avoided. Ice should be applied after the activity. A patellar stabilizing knee brace with a pad about the kneecap in a circular manner should be worn for all activities. Anti-inflammatory medication should be used. The ultimate cure for this problem is appropriate muscle strengthening. By carrying out a quadriceps strengthening program in which the knee is not significantly flexed, the quadriceps will strengthen and help stabilize the kneecap. The best exercises are straight leg raises with an ankle weight and limited arc extensions in which the knee is only brought from approximately 20 degrees of flexion to full extension. Extension exercises and squats in which the knee is brought from the fully flexed to fully extended position should be avoided. If the athlete is not experiencing improvement, orthopaedic evaluation, formal physical therapy, and in rare instances arthroscopy may be required. In some instances, patello-femoral inflammation is due to biomechanical mal alignment of the entire limb and a sports medicine professional may also suggest such corrections as orthotics to realign the feet and legs.

Arthritis is a common problem within the knee joint because it is one of the main weight bearing joints of the body. The onset is usually gradual and without symptoms. In some athletes, injuries to the knee or significant twisting forces can irritate or inflame arthritis which is already present. Arthritis is often described as a constant ache within the knee, but it is usually exacerbated by motion, weight bearing, and activities. It can be present either on the inside or outside portions of the knee, or even in the region behind the kneecap. It can be present in either one or both knees and is usually associated with pain and swelling. Overuse can increase or exacerbate arthritic problems. Rest, ice, and anti-inflammatory medications can decrease the symptoms. Arthritis is diagnosed on physical examination, x-ray, and MRI. If improvement does not occur with these conservative measures, arthroscopic evaluation and smoothing out of the irregular surfaces may be helpful. Physicians may discuss with athletes the fact that if arthritis is present, significant stress and weight bearing on the knee may hasten the worsening of the arthritis present. Avoidance of such activities and relying on less stressful sports such as swimming, golfing, and bike riding versus running and tennis may lessen progression and future problems. Ultimately, if improvement is not seen with conservative measures, a total knee replacement may be indicated.

Bursitis can occur in several regions about the knee. In most cases, it shows up as a relatively painless swelling. In rare cases, infection may be present due to a local cut or abrasion. In instances where significant pain, redness, or warmth are noted, immediate care should be sought. In those instances where a painless swelling is present, one should limit activities, wear a pressure dressing, and use anti-inflammatory medication. This condition often occurs after one has sustained significant chronic pressure to this region or a blow to the front of the knee. In most instances, the swelling will decrease and resolve over several weeks with conservative measures. In rare cases, drainage and injection with corticosteroids may be required by a physician. In extremely rare instances, surgical excision may be needed.

Tendinitis is a common problem about the knee that usually results from an overuse of the various tendons. Many times, this results from flexion and extension activities such as bike riding, swimming, or any sport which involves running. Inflammation can occur in the quadriceps or patellar tendons. It can also occur in the posterior (hamstring) tendons about the knee. It can even occur on the outside of the knee in the ilio-tibial band. Tendinitis usually occurs gradually with motion or activity. Tendinitis is experienced as swelling and tenderness over the tendon involved. It is relieved with rest, ice, and anti-inflammatory medication and ultimately can be prevented and rehabilitated with an aggressive stretching program. If improvement is not felt with conservative measures, the athlete's physician may prescribe injections, physical therapy, or other corrections such as orthotics or changes in one's running style.

LOWER LEG INJURIES

Most lower leg discomforts are due to chronic overuse conditions. Runners and athletes who use running in their sports frequently experience the most problems due to excessive repetitive forces being applied to the lower leg. These injuries can result in either shin splints or stress fractures.

Shin splints stem from excessive stress to the lower inner aspect of the leg where the muscles which act to flex and extend the ankle are attached. Overuse of these muscles can lead to inflammation and discomfort in this area. The pain is usually present after a period of running and will continue for some time afterwards. It is often relieved with rest, but reoccurs with resumed activity. Shoe wear with inadequate support or cushioning may contribute to this condition as well as flat feet. Shin splints may respond to rest, ice, stretching, anti-inflammatory medication, and correction with appropriate foot support including orthotics. In tough cases physical therapy with ultrasound is helpful. Inadequate warming up and stretching is a predisposing factor.

Injuries initially thought to be shin splints may in fact be due to a stress fracture. Instances of discomfort in this region which do not respond to routine care should be medically evaluated, including x-rays. Occasionally, further studies such as a bone scan or MRI may be needed to elucidate stress fractures which result from an excessive repetitive force being applied to the bone over a period of time. Treatment is mainly rest from any repetitive forceful activity to the lower leg. In some instances, non-weight bearing using crutches or even bracing or casting may be required. Recovery usually takes 4 to 8 weeks without any activity followed by gradual resumption of sports.

Other causes of acute discomfort within the leg are strains to the gastroc muscles which are present in the back part of the lower leg. This is often called tennis calf and results from a quick stopping or starting motion. Strains to this area can be either mild or can result in noticeable pain, swelling, and discoloration. If the strain is minor, routine conservative measures can be carried out followed by an aggressive stretching and warmup program with gradual resumption of activities. If the pain and injury is severe, or the discomfort does not quickly resolve, further evaluation should be sought. If warm-ups and stretching are not aggressively added to the athlete's rehabilitation and pre-participation program, there is a high chance of recurrence. Note that this injury is located in the upper part of the lower leg and it needs to be separated from an Achilles tendon rupture which will be discussed below.

ANKLE INJURIES

By far the most common injury sustained about the ankle is that of a sprain. A sprain of the ankle is a stretching or tearing of the ligaments joining the tibia and fibula of the leg to the heel bones of the foot. It almost always results from a twisting injury involving inversion (in) or eversion (out) twisting of the foot on the ankle. It can occur when running on uneven surfaces, when contacting the foot of another player, or even with quickly changing directions and applying irregular forces to the ankle itself.

Ankle sprains can vary in severity. Mild ankle sprains may resolve in several days. Severe ankle sprains may take 8 to 10 weeks for improvement. The more severe sprains result in a complete disruption or tearing of the ligaments either on the inside or outside of the ankle. Ankle sprains show up as an acute injury with swelling, bruising, pain with motion and weight bearing. In certain severe sprains, instability or looseness may also be felt within the ankle. The principles of **RICE** should be acutely applied. If the discomfort and bruising is severe, care should be sought to rule out an ankle fracture. Initial treatment as mentioned includes rest, limited weight bearing on the leg as tolerated, ice, and compression with some kind of a wrap. As the initial injury gradually resolves, the use of a support brace such as an ankle air cast is recommended. Rehabilitation including at least stretching and strengthening exercises and, in many cases, physical therapy are prescribed to speed recovery. Mild sprains may allow the athlete to return to activities in several days. More severe sprains may require casting or bracing and avoidance of athletic activity for up to 8 weeks. If one does not carry out an appropriate rehabilitation program, the ankle may remain somewhat stiff and weak. Incomplete rehabilitation may subject the athlete to recurrent sprains and further problems. In rare instances, the ankle may remain unstable and even require surgery for reconstruction. In other rare instances, continued discomfort and swelling may be present within the ankle due to other injuries, such as a bruising or chipping of the cartilage on the bony structures within the joint. If this occurs, further studies such as an MRI or bone scan may be required along with other treatment, such as arthroscopy.

Ankle fractures result from the same type of injury as ankle sprains. They are usually due to a twisting type of injury. There is significant swelling, pain, and bruising present along with marked discomfort with any weight bearing.

The Achilles tendon is the large tendon in the back part of the ankle and foot which serves to join the posterior calf, gastroc-soleus muscles to the heel or calcaneus. This tendon may be injured acutely in running or sports in which significant forces are applied. In the mature athlete, the Achilles tendon may rupture or tear. This results in marked pain, swelling, and limitation of motion in the ankle. Usually the athlete will be unable to continue with his sport and will have a significant limp. **RICE** should be applied and medical evaluation obtained. Treatment for this injury may be either casting or surgery followed by rehabilitation with physical therapy.

The Achilles tendon may also suffer from overuse and inflammation in the form of a chronic tendinitis. Causes of tendinitis include overuse, lack of stretching, and sometimes biomechanical abnormalities within the feet. The athlete will experience pain about the Achilles which is worse with motion. In some instances, swelling is also present. If Achilles tendinitis continues without improvement, it can eventually lead to weakening and even rupture of the tendon itself. When pain or problems are initially experienced, the activity should be reduced, ice applied, anti-inflammatory medication taken, and aggressive stretching carried out. Sometimes, a heel lift will relieve pressure from the Achilles tendon. When improvement is not forthcoming, a sports medicine evaluation should be obtained.

FOOT INJURIES

The most common problem experienced within the foot in older athletes is that of plantar fasciitis, a.k.a. heel spurs. Plantar fasciitis results from excessive stress being applied to the fascia, or tissue on the bottom surface of the foot. The fascia links the heel to the forefoot and helps create the arch. This structure can become stressed or irritated due to overuse, biomechanical problems within the foot, or improper footwear. Plantar fasciitis is experienced as a chronic injury, felt as a discomfort in the arch of the foot. It is worse with weight bearing and towards the end of the day. Classically, the discomfort is also present within the first ten steps in the morning when getting out of bed. The pain from plantar fasciitis is exacerbated by sporting activity such as sprinting, running on hills, or running on soft surfaces such as sand. Those with flat feet or those who pronate (i.e., roll their foot to the outside) have an increased incidence of plantar fasciitis. Athletes with longstanding plantar fasciitis can develop bone spurs within the front part of the heel, however, this is a secondary phenomenon and not the cause of the problem.

Initial treatment of plantar fasciitis involves cutting back on the offending activity and reassesing one's footwear to make sure that it is relatively new and providing good support. If an athlete is known to have flat feet or a tendency to pronate, shoes with extra stability should be worn. Heel supports or cups which may be obtained in a local pharmacy are also beneficial. Ice will relieve the discomfort and inflammation present. The athlete should work on stretching exercises for the plantar fascia and the Achilles tendon. Anti-inflammatory medication may be helpful. Eventually, strengthening exercises will help prevent future problems. If improvement is not forthcoming within several weeks, evaluation by a professinal may lead to formal physical therapy, a prescription for orthotics, injections, splints to hold the foot in extension at night, and in rare instances even surgery.

Fractures may occur within the foot and can result from direct trauma or from a forceful twisting injury. A common fracture within the foot is that of a Jones fracture. This is a fracture to the fifth metatarsal (pinkie toe) which is located on the outer mid portion of the foot. This injury occurs in the same manner as an ankle sprain. However, the discomfort, swelling, and bruising are within the outside foot and not the ankle. X-rays are required to make this diagnosis and it is usually treated by immobilization with casting. Certain types of Jones fractures have a slow healing rate and, in rare instances, may even require surgery.

Other types of foot fractures which can be experienced are stress fractures. Often, these occur in runners and become obvious as a gradual ache within the foot during and after activity. Stress fractures have point tenderness within the mid portion of the foot. The diagnosis is made with x-ray and/or bone scan. Treatment for a stress fracture is to limit activity including possibly crutches and/or casting. Significant trauma to the foot can lead to numerous other types of fractures and dislocations which require evaluation and are treated individually.

Like other anatomical areas, the foot and ankle can experience arthritis within the numerous joints present, resulting in pain and limitation of motion in the affected area.

As the foot ages, bunions can develop. These present as pain and prominence along the inner aspect of the foot where the great toe joins the mid foot. Bunions are bone spurs associated with angulation of the toes. Initially, shoe wear modification is recommended. In some instances, surgical correction can be quite beneficial. A similar condition can exist on the lateral or outside portion of the foot, this is known as a bunionette. Surgical or conservative treatment is similar to that for bunions.

A specific condition which can exist in the foot is that of a Morton's neuroma. This results from irritation of the digital nerves which exit the foot and progress down the toes providing sensation. These nerves can become irritated between the bony structures at the base of the toes. This inflammation leads to localized discomfort and numbness. Excessively tight footwear is a contributing factor. Initially, rest, wider shoes, and anti-inflammatory medication can be tried. If improvement is not forthcoming, injections and possible surgical treatment is beneficial.

Blisters and callouses are experienced by many senior athletes and those individuals just beginning an exercise program. Both result from excessive friction applied to various parts of the feet. Their formation is related to weight bearing activities. Contributing factors may be shoes that are either too large or too small, excessive moisture, and inappropriate sock materials. Prevention includes keeping the feet dry with frequent sock changes, wearing socks that are of dual layers to keep moisture away from the skin, and appropriately fitting shoes. Distance runners sometimes will lubricate their feet with Vaseline to prevent excessive friction. Blisters are clearly noticeable as fluid collections below the skin. They are frequently painful. In addition to appropriate footwear modifications, the blister should be relieved of pressure and fluid by gently puncturing it with a sterile needle. Then a dressing with a Band-Aid or appropriate material is applied until the blister has healed. In most circumstances, it is ill-advised to remove the separated skin from the surface of the blister.

A callous is an excessive thickening of the skin which is usually present over an area of increased friction or pressure. Again, shoe wear should be checked. The callous may need to be padded to decrease pressure on the area and, in some instances, softened and trimmed with appropriate medical techniques. Callouses can be clues to underlying bony imbalances.

Athletes may experience ingrown toenails in which the corners of the nails will curl and grow into the surrounding skin. This results in significant inflammation and in some cases infection. The incidence of ingrown toenails increases with overly tight shoes and toenails which are trimmed in a curved manner as opposed to a straight transverse direction. Ingrown toenails initially can be treated with warm soaks and avoidance of pressure from shoe wear. In most cases, they should be evaluated by a physician for the addition of anti-biotics and minor surgical excision of the ingrown portion of the nail.

FURTHER GENERAL READING

American Academy of Orthopaedic Surgeons (1991) "Athletic Training in Sports Medicine", Rosemont, IL, 2nd Edition.

Baker, C.L. (1995) The Hughson Clinic Sports Medicine Book, Williams and Wilkins Co., Media, PA

Buckwalter, J.A. (1996) "The Aging Athlete", Sports Medicine and Arthroscopy Review, Vol. 3.

Fu, F.H. and D.A. Stone (1994) Sports Injuries, Williams and Wilkins Co., Baltimore, Maryland.

Taylor, P.M. and D.K. Taylor (1988) "Conquering Athletic Injuries", The American Running and Fitness Association, Leisure Press, Champaign, Illinois.

Chapter

I FIVE

Exercise Training Adaptations in Older Individuals

Exercise training depicts a process of adaptive changes to achieve the strength, power, and cardiorespiratory capacity necessary in order to complete a specific physical task. Endurance training requires several months of rhythmic exercise of a specific frequency, duration, and intensity, which results in an increase in maximal oxygen consumption (VO_2 max), cardiac stroke volume, the number of muscle capillaries, mitochondria, and metabolic enzymes. Strength or resistive exercise training elicits increases in the cross-sectional area of the muscle cells and an increase in their capacity to generate force. Therefore, there are major underlying biochemical changes in the various organs and cells involved in the physical activity that provides the needed energy, strength, and power to carry out specific tasks. Generally speaking, exercise training doesn't convert fast twitch (type II) skeletal muscle to slow twitch (type I), but the fast twitch IIA and IIB fibers do show increases with aerobic and strength training, respectively.

STRENGTH TRAINING

It has been known for a long time that young people in their 20's and 30's can increase their muscle strength with training. In the last 6–8 years it has become obvious that older individuals in the 50's and 60's can increase their strength levels with training as well. In fact, an amazing study carried out in 85–90 year old subjects at a nursing home in Boston has shown that even the oldest individuals can increase their muscle strength and endurance with the proper training.

When the appropriate exercise prescription for strength training is followed for at least 8 to 10 weeks as outlined in Chapter 3, a number of positive changes occur in the skeletal muscles that result in noticeable improvements in muscle strength and endurance. As a result of strength training there is an increase in the size of the individual muscle fibers that ultimately make the whole muscle larger. Put another way, the cross-sectional area or the diameter of the muscle has increased. Normal strength training does not increase the **number** of muscle cells in the trained muscle, only the size of the muscle. The increase in muscle size with training is more noticeable in older men than older women due to gender differences in hormones. However, women do have the capacity to enlarge their muscles with training. This increase in muscle size, which occurs in all the major muscle groups of the upper body and lower body, results in a major improvement in muscle strength. Most individuals who do strength training for 2–4 months will show a 20–40% increase in their strength testing results which varies somewhat with the muscle group tested. Generally speaking, individuals who are weaker and can't lift much weight in the pre-training testing will show the greatest improvement in strength. So if you are small-muscled and have never done strength training before **do not despair**, since you may not be as strong as your friend, partner, or spouse but you may actually make more gains than they do.

In addition to the substantial improvements in muscle strength with strength training, the endurance capacity of the muscles also increases. This means that with training the muscle can contract repeatedly over time before it becomes fatigued. For example, before training the upper arm muscle (biceps, for those human anatomy types) might be able to lift a 10 pound weight 15 times until fatigue sets in. After training, the muscle can contract 30 times lifting the 10 pound weight before tiring, a whopping 100% increase in muscle endurance. The increases in muscle strength and endurance after training have a very practical benefit. Most people find that it is easier to carry out their daily activities after training. That is they are better able to carry the groceries into the house from the car. Lifting chores around the house become less difficult. Perhaps one can work longer and be more productive in the garden during the outdoor season. In the very old who have a hard time climbing stairs, their ability to go up and down stairs improves. There are even several studies that show that strength training can lessen the number of falls in older women and men. Falling is quite common in those over the age of 65 and when folks fall and break a hip or leg, other medical conditions can put them in a serious medical situation.

While strength training is very beneficial for the exercised muscles of the skeleton, this type of training has a minimal effect on the heart muscle and function. Therefore, most exercise physiologists don't recommend strength training as a means to increase cardiovascular fitness. Also, the number of calories burned in strength training types of exercise is quite small so this type of exercise is not the best form of exercise for those individuals who have weight loss as a major goal of their exercise program. The average 30–45 minute weight training exercise session probably burns about 100 calories, i.e., the number of calories in an average slice of bread or large apple. On the other hand, a 30–45 minute aerobic exercise session consisting of walking, jogging, cycling, or stair climbing would burn about 4 times the number of calories of strength training (about 400 calories). But wait! There are some other benefits to strength training as exercise. Strength training has been shown to increase the density of bone in older women and men between the ages of 50 and 75. This is especially so if the exercise training stresses the muscles of the hip, low back, and legs. Ligaments and tendons that attach the muscles to the bones and bones to each other are also stronger after strength training. Recent studies have also suggested that strength training can improve metabolism by reducing the blood sugar (glucose) levels, especially important for those with elevated blood sugars or mild diabetes. Preliminary evidence also indicates that strength training can decrease the time it takes for food to complete its journey through the digestive system, a fact that may help lessen the exposure of cancer causing substances to the system and thereby lower the risk of certain types of cancer. Then, of course, there are more subjective benefits of strength training, like the fact that one feels better after an exercise session, experiences improvement in mood, and benefits from the social aspects of an activity performed with other human beings. Add to this list that one's clothes may fit a bit better and an improvement in outward appearance may become obvious to others, and you have a lot of reasons why a program of regular strength training should be a part of every ones' lifestyle.

AEROBIC TRAINING

It is well known that aerobic training in the form of walking, jogging, cross-country skiing, stair climbing, swimming, roller skating, etc. increases an individual's cardiovascular fitness. This means that the VO_2 max, mentioned in the first chapter as the maximal amount of the oxygen that the body can take in, transfer in the blood, and use in the muscles, is increased. The increase in VO_2 max is usually increased by about 10–25% after several months of training in both men and women.

NEWS FLASH Older individuals in their 50's, 60's, 70's, and right on up to the age of 80, all increase their oxygen transport capacity just as much as young folks in their 20's (remember, you heard it **here** first). What does this mean in practical terms? The improvement in cardiovascular fitness translates into increased capacity to walk and carry out all the activities around the house that use large muscle groups. It may mean an increased ability to climb stairs and even give one the stamina to take a sightseeing tour on foot around our nations capital to see **all** the monuments, not just the Lincoln or the Washington from the bus. Regularly performed aerobic exercise training can increase the length of time that one can perform an activity so that more calories can be burned by the fit person, an obvious advantage to the individual who is interested in losing body fat. There are several physiological mechanisms that lead to this increase in heart function. Number one is the fact that after exercise training the size of the heart increases, so that more blood can be pumped per unit of time. The trained muscles also have a greater ability to absorb oxygen from the blood because there is an increase in the small capillary blood vessels with training. The size and number of the mitochondria (remember the little power house/energy factories in the cell that produce ATP?) also increase, along with the enzymes that help us increase our metabolism. If these weren't enough positive benefits, there is more. Regularly performed aerobic exercise training also lowers the "bad" LDL cholesterol in the blood while raising the "good" HDL's, lowers the level of fat in the blood (triglycerides), and also reduces the sugar or glucose concentration in the blood of those individuals who have elevated blood sugars because of diabetes. Wait, we're not done yet! Exercise training also reduces blood pressure in people who have mild hypertension and increases or prevents the loss of bone in older individuals who may be at risk for osteoporosis. Weight bearing, aerobic exercise is probably best for optimal bone health, activities like walking/jogging and stair climbing put the greatest stress on the tendons and bones thus leading to an increase in bone mineral density.

The benefits of strength training and aerobic training are many, while the risks are few. The benefits are there for older individuals to acquire since they respond to exercise training just as well as young folks do, as long as the intensity, frequency, duration, and progression of the exercise is well-suited to the fitness level of the participant. Probably the best plan of action for older people is to combine a program of regular aerobic and strength training to fit their current lifestyle.

FURTHER GENERAL READING

Anderson K.L. (1968). The Cardiovascular System in Exercise. In Exerc. Phys. H.B. Falls, editor, Academic Press, New York, USA.

Klug G.A. and Tibbits G.F. (1988). The Effect of Activity on Calcium Mediated Entry in Striated Muscle. Exerc. Sports Sci. Rev. 16:1–59.

McArdle W.D. et. al (1996). Exercise Physiology. 4th Edition, pp. 1–853. Lea & Febiger, Philadelphia (USA).

Powers, S.K. And E.T. Howley. (1994) Exercise Physiology: Theory and Application to Fitness and Performance. Brown and Benchmark, 2nd Edition, Dubuque, IA, pp. 263–284.

Saltin B. et. al. (1977). Fiber Types and Metabolic Potentials of Skeletal Muscles in Sedentary Man and Endurance Runners. Ann. N.Y. Acad. Sci., 301:3–29.

Wilmore J.H. and Costill D.L. (1988). Training For Sport and Activity, 3rd Edition, pp. 1–420, Wm. C. Brown Publishers, Dubuque, Iowa (USA).

Chapter
SIX

Physical Activity and Longevity

Science has showed us that the maximum life span in humans has not changed appreciably and probably will not in the immediate future. However, modern medical technology and increased attention to lifestyle habits such as exercise, proper nutrition, optimal body weight status, and the avoidance of certain unhealthy behaviors has increased the number of individuals living to an older age, i.e., longevity is increased. A second issue has to do with the quality of that extended life. Are older individuals capable of taking care of themselves, enjoying their independence and the ability to follow their favorite recreational activities? The answer is not always yes to this question, but it does appear that those individuals who remain active and participate in regular physical activity have an enhanced quality of life.

QUANTITY OF LIFE

If the aging process could be slowed down, human beings could live longer; and if the process could be stopped, people could live forever. Based on current scientific knowledge, it is not possible to stop the aging process and it is probably true that we will always age and die. The maximum documented life span for our human species is about 110 years of age and this will continue to be so for the future as far, as we can see. The **average** life span, on the other hand, is about 85 years of age and it is well known this number has been increasing from the early 1900's due to improvements in medical treatment, decreases in harmful pollutants in the environment, reductions in the rates of smoking/drinking/drug abuse, declines in the rates of violent crime, and the increase in the willingness of people to make healthy lifestyle changes.

Longevity refers to the number of individuals who live longer than the average life span for the particular species. Most of the aging studies dealing with maximum life span and longevity have been conducted in laboratory rats because they are easier to study over a life span of 3 years rather than 70 or 80 years, as in humans. The animal studies show that one of the only treatments that are effective in slowing the rate of aging is food restriction. These studies are carried out in such a way where one group of animals is allowed to eat as much food as they want and the other group is fed a nutrient complete diet but it has 30% fewer calories than the freely eating animals. The animals on the food restricted diet live significantly longer than the freely eating animals. Alas, food restriction has not been shown to have the same effect on the rate of aging in humans.

Physical activity in animals has also been found to have an affect on aging. In these studies, control sedentary animals who have no access to exercise are compared with animals housed in cages that have running wheels attached to the side so that the animals can run in the wheels whenever they feel like it. The physically active animals don't live longer than the sedentary ones, that is the life span is not increased, but many more of the animals who exercise reach a certain old age. So, in animals physical activity has a positive effect on longevity.

What about in our favorite species, human beings? Human experiments also show that physically active individuals live longer than sedentary folks. A 1978 study showed that track athletes live longer than non-athletes. A 1990 study in the Netherlands showed that when highly fit male ice skaters who did long distance skating were studied over 32 years, they had a longer life expectancy than the average population in the country. The best physical activity and longevity study that has been conducted is the Harvard Alumni Study that was published in 1986. The researchers studied over 16,000 Harvard graduates aged 35–74 who were asked to fill out health history and physical activity questionaires. Physical activity was measured as the number of calories expended per week for the subjects. The men who expended at least 2,000 calories per week in addition to their minimum weekly caloric requirements (the equivalent of 4–5 hours of brisk walking or jogging) had a 30% lower death rate than the men who exercised less. The effects of the exercise were calculated to have extended the lives of the active alumni by about 2 years. Of course, the wise guy comedians and other syndicated humor columnists, we won't mention any names (Dave Barry!) reacted to this study when it first came out by saying it's great to get an extra couple of years of life but it was "wasted by having to spend it trudging on a treadmill or sweating on a stationary bicycle." All of the preceding has been a description of the effects of physical activity and exercise on the **quantity** of life. But is that all that should be considered?

QUALITY OF LIFE

The factors listed in Table 3 summarize those components of our existence that directly affect the quality of life for older, and even very old individuals. Out of the 5 major listings in the table, exercise and physical activity have an impact on 4 of these factors. It is well known that exercise has an anti-depressant effect on people, in fact, many psychiatrists and psychologists prescribe exercise for their patients who suffer clinical depression. There is the exercise "high" type of feeling that many people experience during and after physical activity

Table 6.1. Factors affecting the Quality of Life

- Emotional Function and Feelings of Well Being
- Cognitive Function
- Economic Status
- Social and Recreational Activities
- Health Status, Energy, Vitality, and Physical Function

(the runner's high), as well as the fact that exercise improves self-esteem in many people by making them feel good about themselves. There is a sense of accomplishment in performing physical work or exercise, plus the fact that people feel satisfaction about doing sometime good for themselves. Recent studies show that exercise and aerobic training in older people may be able to increase the ability to process information in the central nervous system, thereby having an effect on the efficiency of cognitive function. Many a writer, painter, or scientist will mention that they have their most productive thinking and creating sessions after having performed some exercise. Physical activity and exercise training sessions also provide for a social outlet, especially if one goes to a fitness facility or joins friends on a regular basis. This is not only a physical time but a social one too. Many friendships have been cultivated and maintained over years through exercise. An example is the squash players who meet at the gym at our university every Tuesday and Thursday for years to play the game they love. There is also a running club for over 40 year old master runners who meet every Saturday morning at the Washington Sailing Marina near National Airport in Washington, D.C. to run and socialize together. They have done this for over 20 years. The exercise has become a social activity that is cherished and at the same time, the social nature of the activity has kept the participants active for a long time. Last, but certainly not least, is the fact that exercise has the effect of improving health status and physiological function.

Cardiovascular fitness and muscle strength and endurance translate into an increased ability to carry out the activities of daily living such as walking, food preparation, personal health care, work around the house, lifting, writing, and the like. It is all these activities, plus the ability to get out and be mobile that contribute to an active quality of life.

To summarize, physical activity and exercise training have a positive effect on both the quantity and quality of life in older individuals.

FURTHER GENERAL READING

Katch, F.I. and W.D. McArdle (1993) Aging, Exercise, and Cardiovascular Health. In: Introduction to Nutrition, Exercise, and Health. Lea and Febiger, Philadelphia, 4th Edition, pp. 363–387.

Paffenbarger, R.S., Jr. et al. (1986) Physical Activity, all-cause mortality, and longevity of college alumni. *N. Engl. J. Med.* 314:605–612.

Spirduso, W.W. Issues of Quantity and Quality of Life. In: Physical Dimensions of Aging, Human Kinetics Publishers, Champaign, IL, pp. 5–29, 1995.

Chapter

I SEVEN

Temperature Regulation During Exercise in Older People

Water is the most important nutrient for an individual before, during, and after exercise. During exercise, all of the energy expenditure leads to a large amount of heat production. Evaporation of water through the skin (i.e., sweating) is the critical avenue for cooling and maintaining the core body temperature. In older individuals, sweating and blood circulation are diminished with aging. These two factors contribute to diminished heat tolerance. The evaporated water which is lost during exercise should be replenished in order to restore the normal blood and cellular ionic concentrations which are vital to normal functions. In addition, drinking cold water can cool the body and maintain it at 37°C. Older persons should drink 1–2 glasses of cold water two hours prior to an exercise session to promote hydration and allow for

the excretion of excess fluid. Also, older people should
drink 1 glass of water for every 1 lb of weight loss during
exercise. During exercise, the person should drink 4–6
ounces of water every 15–20 minutes to insure proper
hydration. If the body temperature is not maintained at
37°C, the following heat-related illnesses (in order of
increasing seriousness) can occur: heat cramps, heat
exhaustion, and heat stroke.

Water is the most critical nutrient for the survival and well
being of a person. One can survive without the intake of other
nutrients for days, weeks, and even months, but cannot
survive without water for more than a few days. In a young,
70 kg (154 lb) person, the water content is about 40 liters (i.e.,
60% of body weight). However, as we age, the water content
decreases to about 50% of body weight. Therefore, the water
content of a 70 year old person can be as low as 35 liters. Most
of the water (22 liters) is inside cells; nevertheless, about
13 liters reside outside of cells.

The blood volume is about 4.4 liters and the maintenance of
this volume is critical to a person's survival, despite the fact
that daily fluid intake can vary from 1–8 liters. Excess fluid
intake can easily be regulated; however, a problem arises
when fluid intake is below one liter per day and blood
volume starts to decrease below 4.4 liters (for example, a
blood volume of less than 4 liters can cause death). Under
sedentary conditions, the skin (via evaporation) and the
kidneys (via urine output) are the most important regulators
of body water. Under conditions of hot weather and exercise
(despite fluid intake in many cases), the skin becomes the only
important regulator of body water and body temperature.
Loss of water in a heavy, prolonged bout of exercise (e.g., a
3 hour marathon) can increased from 0.1 to 5 liters, a very
substantial loss indeed.

HEAT TOLERANCE IN OLDER INDIVIDUALS

Sweating, where heat is lost from the skin via evaporation, is
an absolute necessity in maintaining constant body tempera-

ture. The sweat rate in exercising humans usually corresponds to increases in energy expenditure by the athlete. Some discussion exists as to whether older persons lose their ability to acclimatize and adapt to exercise heat stress. Early studies did show that less fit older persons did have higher heart rates under heat stress, compared with their more fit and younger counterparts. Comparative studies in fit young and old runners show no difference in heat responses to marathon running. The very famous physiologist, D.B. Dill, showed that the capacity for sweating is sufficient to maintain body temperature in 50–84 year subjects during prolonged desert walks. Thus, as long as physical fitness, age, body size and composition, and state of acclimatization are taken into account there doesn't appear to be much loss of heat tolerance with aging that affects temperature regulation.

Having said this, one should also realize that it has been shown that with aging there is a delayed onset of sweating and a reduction in the output of the sweat glands. Furthermore, older athletes show a 25–40% reduction in skin blood flow and a reduced thirst drive after exercise, which may mean that older persons do not recover from exercise in the heat as rapidly and may place themselves in a chronic state of dehydration during the warm months of the year spent exercising. This chronic decrease in fluid volume of the blood could impair the temperature regulation of older athletes and persons exercising in the heat. Fluid losses during adult baseball games can range from 1% to 3% of body weight. Obviously, such a loss should be dealt with in a more serious manner in older athletes than younger ones. It is more common to not recognize dehydration in older individuals, and this is especially true if the older individual suffers from an illness that causes fever, diarrhea, or vomiting.

FLUID STATUS

Some of the energy expenditure during exercise results in heat production, mostly by the active skeletal muscle. Therefore, body temperature will rise rapidly during exercise if cooling due to sweating does not occur. The prolonged increase in

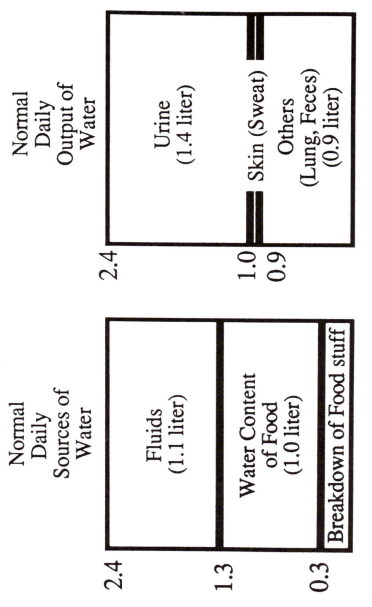
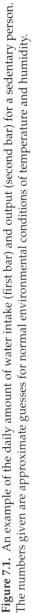

Figure 7.1. An example of the daily amount of water intake (first bar) and output (second bar) for a sedentary person. The numbers given are approximate guesses for normal environmental conditions of temperature and humidity.

body temperature will eventually cause serious damage to the thermo-regulatory system, which can result in serious damage to the body's most sensitive organ, the brain. Also, even moderate dehydration could contribute to changes in mental status and may increase the risk of muscle injury. Thirst, unfortunately, is not a reliable indicator of water loss or rise in body temperature during exercise, especially in older persons. Therefore, older athletes and recreational exercisers should drink water or other fluid not just to quench their thirst, but as part of their exercise regime. Figures 7.1 and 7.2 represent a hypothetical daily water output and water intake for people who are sedentary, who have run a 3 hour marathon, or are

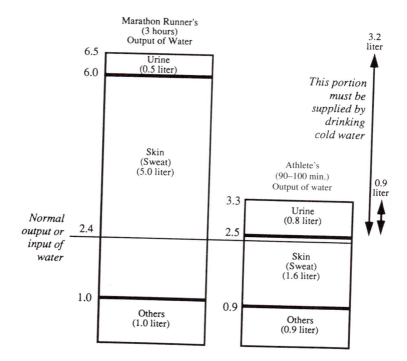

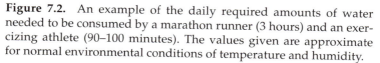

Figure 7.2. An example of the daily required amounts of water needed to be consumed by a marathon runner (3 hours) and an exercizing athlete (90–100 minutes). The values given are approximate for normal environmental conditions of temperature and humidity.

exercising (90–100 minutes). The numbers are rough estimates, and are only for illustrative purposes. The most scientific way to determine optimal water intake is to weigh the person before and during the event. The loss of weight due to water loss should be adjusted by drinking the same amount of water. Remember, it is better to drink more than less water. In fact, the American College of Sports Medicine recommends that exercisers drink as much fluid as is comfortably possible. The older person should drink 1–2 glasses of water two hours before the event and 1 glass of water for every 1 lb weight loss during the event. Alternatively, the master athlete or older exerciser could do well by simply drinking 4–6 ounces of water every 15–20 minutes during the event. The water should be cold for two reasons: cold water provides a greater capacity to lower core body temperature and it quickens the emptying of the stomach content into the intestines where water absorption occurs. Also, most people prefer cold/cool fluid to drink. Another factor that increases the desire to drink fluid (i.e., palatability) is whether or not the fluid is flavored or sweetened. Experiments have shown that flavored and/or sweetened beverages will increase the amount of fluid ingested and therefore help to offset the loss of fluid via sweating.

Electrolytes such as Na^+ (sodium/salt), K^+ (potassium), Cl^- (chloride), Ca^{2+} (calcium), and Mg^{2+} (magnesium) are very important ions and their concentrations in the cell and blood are critical for maintaining normal body function. As we sweat more during exercise, the amount of these ions in the sweat is less than that of the blood. In other words, the body is losing more water than ions. Under heavy exercise conditions, the body loses about 5–7 grams of sodium. However, there is a minimal loss of K^+ and Mg^{2+}. Under conditions of continued exercise (up to 60 minutes) there is a need to replenish water continuously, but not sodium. If there is heavy exercise beyond 60 minutes, sodium and carbohydrate replenishment is appropriate. Two to four glasses of about 6% carbohydrate solution is recommended. The use of salt tablets during the early phase of exercise (as in most cases of exercise in older individuals) is detrimental to the body's thermo-regulatory system. The body fluid has a higher salt concentration after exercise than before; therefore, the body's cells need pure water to bring the blood composition back to normal levels. The presence of sodium in drinking water may slightly facilitate water absorption through the intestines and its retention in the body, but only if there has been little sodium in the diet from previous meals. While it may be true that sodium replacement is needed in very prolonged bouts of exercise that last for many hours, "sport drinks" advocates (primarily companies that sell them) promote drinking "sport drinks" for rehydration. For older endurance athletes who are performing 2–3 hour bouts of exercise or for athletic competitions lasting this long, persons should consume beverages with 4–8% carbohydrate content (most sports drinks have this composition). However, since the health risks from dehydration far outweigh the risks taken because of a small amount of salt depletion (not present in most limited activities), it is therefore of paramount importance to first ensure proper hydration with water and carbohydrate if the exercise is of long duration.

After the bout of exercise, the individual should ingest large amounts of carbohydrates in order to replenish muscle glycogen content. The ingestion of carbohydrates within the first two hours after the event is preferred because it is at this time that muscles have an enhanced capacity to synthesize glycogen. Calcium supplementation maybe needed especially for female athletes if blood calcium levels are low. Both older men and women tend not to tolerate low dietary calcium, which is probably due to lower absorption. Therefore, it is recommended that older individuals should consume 800 mg of calcium daily either from food, supplements, or both.

HEAT INJURY AND ILLNESS

Aging athletes may have an added vulnerability to heat related injuries, especially if they routinely exercise for long periods of time in warm and humid climates. The following are heat-related conditions that can occur when exercising in the heat. Athletes and those individuals supervising athletes or recreational exercisers should be mindful of the symptoms of heat illness as outlined in the following section of this chapter.

HEAT CRAMPS

Cause: Heat cramps feel similar to other muscle cramps, like a knot or "charley horse," and may be due to increases in muscle temperature, dehydration, fatigue, lack of blood supply, etc. Reduced blood flow to the muscle due to loss of water, fatigue, prolonged loss of minerals, etc.

Symptoms: Spasmodic tonic contraction of a given muscle (e.g., abdominal and extremities) During exercise usually in the calf or hamstring on the back of the thigh or the quads on the front of the thigh.

Onset: Gradual or sudden.

Danger: None if treated. Heat cramps could result in a termination of that particular exercise for a few days.

Prevention: Regular exercise training in a hot environment, proper warm-up and stretching exercises prior to the activity. Proper hydration before, during, and after the exercise. Sometimes heat cramps in the legs can be relieved with a steady stretching exercise or light massage of the affected muscle.

Treatment: Termination of activity. Stretching, rest, and ice treatment.

HEAT EXHAUSTION

Cause: Loss of water.

Symptoms: Tiredness, malaise, progressive weakness, anxiety, dizziness, fainting, and hot/dry skin. Persons will experience sweating, a small urine volume, and perhaps unconsciousness.

Onset: Gradual; over several days.

Danger: Rarely, the athlete may go into shock because of reduced blood volume. However, typically heat exhaustion is not an emergency condition. If not treated, this illness can lead to heat stroke.

Prevention: Proper/gradual acclimatization to exercise in the heat and proper hydration before and during exercise.

Treatment: Termination of activity, rest in a recumbent position in a cool place, drinking water, and later drinking large amounts of mineral rich fluid such as diluted (1:3) fruit and vegetable juices.

HEAT STROKE

Background: Brain cells in the hypothalamus maintain body temperature close to 37°C (98.6). These cells respond to the blood temperature that passes through them. The cells regulate body temperature by sending signals to release skin vasodilators in order to increase sweating. When rectal temperatures reach 41–43°C, unconsciousness may occur; if that happens, the mortality rate ranges from 50–70%. Heat stroke is the second biggest cause of death after accidental death among athletes. In a recent August 1996 story, 14 Mexican troops died in training exercise (The Washington Post, August 3, 1996, p. A24).

Cause: Loss of water and a sudden, uncontrolled rise in body temperature due to the failure of the thermo-regulatory center in the brain.

Symptoms: Heat stroke should be treated as a life threatening medical emergency, as it may lead to death or irreversible brain damage. The person shows behavioral or mental status changes during heat stress. These symptoms include a sense of impending doom, headache, dizziness, confusion, hysteria, and weakness. The person exhibits hot and dry skin, rapid pulse, and low blood pressure.

Factors which could lead to heat stroke include:

a. environmental high temperature and high humidity.

b. high rectal temperature.

    c. hot dry skin (i.e., sweating stops).

    d. cardiorespiratory (e.g., rapid/weak pulse, low blood pressure) and central nervous system disturbances.

    e. clouded consciousness and finally, collapse.

Onset: Sudden.

Danger: Brain damage and death is imminent if not treated quickly.

Prevention: Proper physical fitness and proper hydration before and during exercise.

Heat Illness Chart

Heat Stress

(Environmental high temperature and heavy exercise)

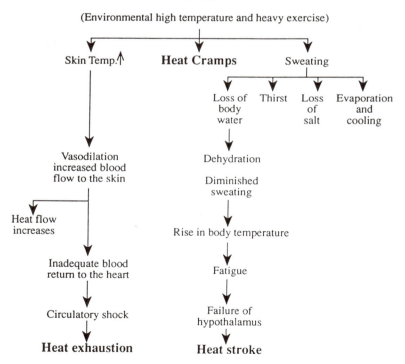

Figure 7.3. Flowchart of heat related illnesses and the relevant pathways that lead to heat cramps, heat exhaustion, and heat stroke.

Treatment:

1. Call for an ambulance.

2. Remove clothes and cool with ice and cold water on the body.

3. Monitor vital signs. (i.e., breathing, heart beat, pupil size).

4. Massage extremities to promote cooling.

5. Once the body temperature cools and the person is quite alert, remove from cold environment to prevent hypothermia.

6. Do not attempt to force water on an unconscious individuals as they will choke on it.

Figure 7.3 represents a flow diagram which summarizes how the various heat related illnesses can result from heat stress. It is important for supervisory persons to realize that once an older person or athlete undergoes a bout of heat exhaustion or heat stroke, he/she may have damaged their thermo-regulatory system. The thermo-regulatory system has a set point of 37°C, but the damaged thermo-regulatory system may have a higher set point and thus the athlete may become more susceptible to bouts of heat related illness, and can further damage the thermo-regulatory system. Therefore, it is important for the athlete to exercise preventive measures in order to reduce the chances of heat related illness.

FURTHER GENERAL READING

Barr S.I. et al. (1990). Fluid Replacement During Prolonged Exercise: Effects of Water, Saline, or No Fluid. Med. Sci. Sports Exerc. 23:811–817.

Coyle E.F. et al. (1983). Carbohydrate Feeding During Prolonged Strenuous Exercise Can Delay Fatigue. J. of Appl. Phys. 55:230–235.

American College of Sport Medicine (1996), Position Stand, "Exercise and Fluid Replacement", Med. Sci. Sports Exerc., 28:i–vii.

Oxford Textbook on Sports Medicine (1994), edited by Haries et al., Oxford Medical Publications, pp. 1–748.

Chapter

EIGHT

Nutritional Concerns for Exercise in Older People

The most beneficial diet for an older person, whether exercising or not, involves eating balanced meals where about 55–60% of the calories come from carbohydrates, 20–25% of the calories from fat, and about 20–25% from protein. Healthy dietary practices for older, exercising individuals are essential because they may be at risk of poor nutritional habits. This may expose older individuals to nutritional deficiencies during heavy bouts of exercise and inhibit recuperation from illness, serious injury, or an operation. When exercising, the body requires additional calories, and the best source of these calories for an athlete is from carbohydrates. In general, this means that the diet should include an increase in the percentage of calories from carbohydrates. Pre-event meals should be primarily composed of carbohydrates, and balanced meals should be eaten for several days prior to the event. Just prior to and during the exercise, the athlete should drink adequate amounts of cold water (2–3 glasses). In an ideal situation, the athlete should drink 4–6 ounces of water every 15–20 minutes during the event. Since calcium has been shown to be an important mineral in the formation of bone as well as in preventing loss of bone with aging, it has been suggested recently that older women and men increase the daily intake of calcium via the foods that they eat or by supplements so that receive at least 1,200 mg a day.

BASIC NUTRITIONAL PLAN

The human body is an organism composed of cells that have certain nutritional requirements that are needed to maintain normal cell function so that the various metabolic processes essential to life are carried out. Like the average American, many athletes, trainers, and coaches have a very limited knowledge of nutrition and the metabolic basis of exercise and training. Unfortunately, societal pressures and the "win at all cost" mentality induces athletes and those who coach them to invent or subscribe to many bizarre concoctions of food or supplements to enhance performance, which are then deemed proper "nutrition." Many of these wild recipes and diet plans are not based on scientific studies but on the testimony of successful athletes, coaches, and those who sell various products to earn money. Most of these recipes are based on personal experiences associated with the food last eaten before a successful performance. Currently, there are no recommended daily allowances (RDAs as the nutritionists call them) for carbohydrate and fat in the diet. However, an older athlete or individual performing regular exercise training should maintain a balanced diet consisting of three main constituents: carbohydrates (55–60% of calories), fats (20–25%), and protein (about 20%) (See Table 8.1). Nutritionists suggest about 1 gram of protein in your diet for each kilogram of body weight. For an average older person who weighs about 175 pounds this means approximately 80 grams of protein per day. For example, eighty grams of protein would be found in the following: two 8 oz. glasses of skim milk, one 8 oz. cup of

Table 8.1. Estimated Amount of Carbohydrates, Proteins, and Fats an Older Athlete Should Ingest Daily

	Average activity		Endurance activity (2-hr skiing session*)	
	Athlete's weight		Athlete's weight	
	55 kg (121 lb)	70 kg (154 lb)	55 kg (121 lb)	70 kg (154 lb)
Carbohydrate (g)	315–630	400–600	415–715	520–720
Proteins (g)	60–70	80–90	60–70	80–90
Fats (g)	60–80	80–100	60–80	80–10

*It is estimated that a 1-hr intense exercise session consumes 400 calories.

non-fat yogurt, a 6 oz. turkey and low fat cheese sandwich on whole wheat bread, and a 2 oz. of soybeans on a medium dinner salad (or several oz. of nuts).

Unfortunately, the current average American diet is composed of about 40+ % of the calories from fat, too much protein, and not enough complex carbohydrates (the kind of carbohydrates found in unrefined grains, pasta, rice, potatoes, fruits, etc. The Heart Healthy Diet, as advocated by the American Heart Association, is one where less than 30% of one's daily calories come from fat and only 10% of the fat calories come from saturated fat (oils, margarines, meat, etc.) Healthy and balanced nutritional intake by the individual will not only help the older athlete but also will diminish the chances of developing coronary heart disease and becoming obese.

Older individuals, because of age, inactivity, economics, becoming homebound, or stress may be at a high risk of poor nutrition due to an inadequate diet. Therefore, older individuals may be at an even greater risk of malnutrition when faced with a significant physical or emotional stress, or when recuperating from illness, injury, or operation. It is for these reasons that the nutritional intake of older active and sedentary individuals is very, very important for their overall health status.

ENERGY SOURCES

The immediate source of energy for muscle activity within each cell is a chemical molecule called adenosine triphosphate (ATP). Muscle action is an organized composite of the action of individual cells. ATP is an intracellular substance which contains three phosphate molecules, and it is through the breakdown of the terminal phosphate that energy is produced. The amount of ATP available in each cell is very small, and only provides sufficient energy to last less than 1–2 seconds in an exhaustive sprint-like exercise. However, the cell attempts to maintain a fairly constant level of ATP, especially during moderate activities. The substance which helps to provide an immediate source of ATP is the molecule phosphocreatine (also called creatine phosphate, PCr). PCr phosphorylates (i.e., adds one phosphate) adenosine diphosphate (ADP) to form ATP. However, the amount of ATP and PCr combined lasts less than about 10 seconds in an exhaustive exercise. The long range source of energy for the cell comes from two main processes that involve utilizing the energy stored in foodstuffs. These two processes are:

1. **Glycolysis.** ATP is produced anaerobically (without oxygen) from sugar derived from stored muscle glycogen. Glycogen is a polysaccharide (i.e., it consists of many sugars) molecule consisting of hundreds to thousands of glucose molecules linked together. Anaerobic exercise produces lactic acid which can accumulate and have adverse effects on performance. However, the anaerobic process does provide ATP when the body needs it as a quick source of energy (i.e., for sprint-like exercise).

2. **Oxidation.** ATP is produced aerobically (with oxygen) from carbohydrates, fats, and proteins. The aerobic oxidation process produces 13 times more ATP for the same amount of starting material than ATP which is anaerobically produced by glycolysis. While the aerobic process is slow, it provides long lasting energy for exercises such as jogging and marathon running.

Figure 8.1 gives a hypothetical order of the utilization of energy in a bout of activity. Cellular ATP and ATP derived from phosphorylation by PCr are utilized first. Individuals simultaneously use the anaerobic and the aerobic systems as the situation demands.

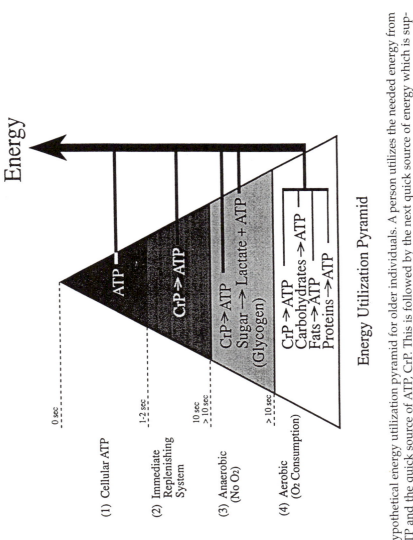

Energy Utilization Pyramid

Figure 8.1. A hypothetical energy utilization pyramid for older individuals. A person utilizes the needed energy from the available ATP and the quick source of ATP, CrP. This is followed by the next quick source of energy which is supplied by the anaerobic process – this is for when the individual engages in bursts of activities. The long range source of energy for an individual is derived through aerobic processes.

A well trained person has an advantage over the untrained person in the utilization of energy. In another chapter, we describe in detail the biochemical changes due to training. However, we will briefly describe the physiological and biochemical advantages of a trained individual in utilizing the energy pyramid of figure 8.1.

In a trained individual, the levels of ATP and PCr are higher and thus last about 20–30% longer than in an untrained person. More importantly, the trained person has a greater glycolytic capacity (almost twice as much) as the untrained person. Furthermore, the aerobic system (i.e., enzymes, substrates, etc.) is also more efficiently developed in the trained person. The trained person can therefore produce ATP faster for the aerobic exercises needed during the activity. Above all, the trained person can recover sooner from a bout of exercise because of the increased levels of enzymes, substrates and capacity to produce ATP.

LACTATE AND FATIGUE

The breakdown of ATP to produce energy results in the production of a hydrogen ion, and thus lowers the cellular pH. This intracellular change in pH eventually lowers the blood's pH. The presence of hydrogen ions is normally a signal for the respiratory system and kidneys to get rid of the excess hydrogen ions. However, under stressful conditions hydrogen ions and/or lactate can accumulate; eventually, the build up of these molecules may contribute to muscle fatigue. Trained individuals physiologically adapt in such a way which allows them to be able to perform adequately in the presence of higher lactate blood levels. Moreover, trained individuals tend to utilize and dissipate lactate better than the untrained person. In older persons, lactate dissipation is less efficient due to less efficient circulation. Therefore, lactate removal requires longer periods after exercise to eliminate lactate. The specificity of training for a given sport is important in adapting the tissues to those stressful conditions of the given sport in order to stimulate cellular mechanisms of adaptation to those conditions.

CARBOHYDRATES

Carbohydrates are composed of carbon, hydrogen, and oxygen. The simplest form of carbohydrate is the sugar glucose. Other examples of simple carbohydrates are fructose and galactose. Examples of some complex carbohydrates are starch (e.g., from potatoes) and cellulose (a source of dietary fiber). The average American currently consumes 50% of carbohydrates as simple sugars, mainly in the form of sucrose. However, sucrose causes a fluctuation in insulin secretion. Too much insulin in the blood may lead to low blood sugar (hypoglycemia). Low blood sugar could contribute to symptoms such as weakness, dizziness, and hunger sensations. None of these symptoms are beneficial to the athlete during their activities. Dizziness in older individuals needs to be avoided because it can contribute to injuries (e.g., bone) through mishaps. Fructose (fruit sugar) is absorbed well in the intestine and does not stimulate insulin secretion. Thus it does not promote large fluctuations in blood sugar levels. As we have mentioned earlier, exercise suppresses insulin secretion. Therefore, sugar intake during exercise will not lead to low blood sugar.

Carbohydrates serve as the main source of energy for the brain and during exercise when the exercise intensity is very high. Carbohydrate in the form of blood glucose and glucose that is released from stored glycogen in the muscles and liver contribute to our ability to perform intense exercise like sprinting for several laps on an outdoor track or cycling very fast for 2–3 minutes or swimming 2 lengths of the pool all out.

How Does Carbohydrate Improve Our Metabolism?

PROTEIN SPARING

Proteins, as we will see later, are the main building blocks needed for muscle maintenance and repair in older individuals. Proteins can also serve as a source of energy when carbohydrates are low. When needed, glucose is actually formed from proteins as is the case in marathon running or any other prolonged exercise (greater than 90 minutes). Under these conditions, muscle proteins are degraded in order to provide a source of glucose. This actually causes a reduction in muscle content and in the process increases the concentration of nitrogen (from the degradation of proteins) excreted in the urine. Therefore, the maintenance of an adequate supply of carbohydrates or body stores of carbohydrates in the form of glycogen is very important in reducing muscle breakdown in older individuals. This is especially true if tissues are subjected to trauma where repair needs are high, which produces an additional burden for proteins.

CARBOHYDRATES AS A PRIMER FOR FAT UTILIZATION

Carbohydrates in the body undergo metabolism (i.e., breakdown to smaller units) in order to release useful energy. Some of the breakdown products of carbohydrates are needed to break down fats and release their energy. Therefore, when insufficient carbohydrates exist, fatty acid breakdown becomes incomplete and results in acidic body fluids; this is not conducive for normal function.

CARBOHYDRATES AS A SOURCE OF FUEL FOR THE BRAIN

The brain (i.e., central nervous system) utilizes glucose almost solely as its source of energy. Under low carbohydrate conditions, the brain utilizes larger amounts of fats as a source of energy. Nevertheless, low blood glucose due to even modestly low carbohydrate levels could cause the symptoms of hypoglycemia mentioned earlier, and under extreme conditions could even cause irreversible brain damage. However, the brain can adapt by using fats as a source of energy within a week of experiencing low blood sugar.

EXERCISE AND STORED ENERGY

Glucose and carbohydrates are the most likely sources of energy when there is an immediate demand, such as in anaerobic exercise (e.g., sprinting). However, endurance sports are aerobic in nature and they utilize the most efficient forms of metabolism (using oxygen) to break down sugar and carbohydrates which are then used as energy sources.

A carbohydrate-rich diet results in increased stores of muscle and liver glycogen. About 75% of glycogen is usually stored in muscle, 20% in the liver, and the remainder is stored elsewhere. Glycogen stores are the critical factor that determine how long an athlete can exercise before becoming exhausted. There is a near linear relationship between the length of time an athlete can sustain an exercise and the amount of stored glycogen that is used. The ingestion of glucose polymers (series of glucose molecules hooked together) during exercise can prolong the exercise time to exhaustion. Moreover, glucose-polymers do not decrease the transit time of food in the intestine. The decrease in transit time in intestine would decrease absorption of the glucose-polymer. After an event, the athlete has low levels of muscle glycogen. Therefore, it is advisable for the athlete to ingest large quantities of carbohydrates within the first two hours after the event. The muscle content of glycogen is very low following an event and thus there is an enhanced ability in the muscle to store glycogen. Since the glycogen storage enzymes work much more efficiently after exercise, it is important that the athlete takes advantages of this enhanced proficiency by ingesting a large amount of carbohydrates after the event. In this way, the athlete will build up an adequate store of carbohydrates which can then be utilized at subsequent games. Obviously, adequate rest and proper food intake must accompany exercise.

PROTEINS

Proteins consist of carbon, oxygen, hydrogen, and nitrogen. Nitrogen is the distinct atom that is associated with proteins as compared to fats and carbohydrates which only consist of carbon, oxygen, and hydrogen. Also, proteins may contain sulfur, phosphorus, and iron. Proteins, which are large molecules made up of smaller molecules called amino acids, are required for numerous bodily functions. Among the most important body functions that involves proteins are enzymatic processes; transport; storage; the delivery of small molecules such as iron (Fe^{2+}), sodium (Na^+), potassium (K^+), calcium (Ca^{2+}) etc; muscle function (e.g., in skeletal and heart muscle); mechanical support (e.g., collagen in fibers); the immune system (all antibodies against foreign invaders are proteins); nerve function (e.g., many neurotransmitters are proteins); and growth and differentiation (e.g., hormones, regulation of genes, etc). There are nine amino acids (called essential amino acids) which are not synthesized in the adult body, and must be provided through the intake of foods. The other eleven amino acids are synthesized in the body and thus need not be provided by a food source. These are called non-essential amino acids. The most important sources of proteins are meat, fish, poultry, eggs, and dairy products.

At the beginning of each heavy training season, serious older athletes should increase their intake of proteins by almost 20–30%. This increased protein intake will compensate for the immediate need to increase muscle mass, and other amino acid-requiring proteins such as red blood cells and myoglobin (the oxygen carrier in muscle). As we have mentioned earlier, it has been observed that prolonged exercise causes protein breakdown when carbohydrate reserves are low. In older athletes this is highly undesirable since aging and/or inactivity is associated with loss of muscle mass. Therefore, an athlete should have an abundance of glycogen stores in the muscle in order to prevent muscle wastage and to maintain peak performance levels. Glycogen stores are replenished by the intake of a sufficient amount of carbohydrates.

FATS

Fats, like carbohydrates, also consist of carbon, oxygen, and hydrogen. Also, fats may contain phosphorous, nitrogen, and other elements. Fats are required for numerous bodily functions; among the most important are energy stores (i.e., fats produce the energy currency of the body, ATP); structure (e.g., all cell membranes are made of fats); hormones (some are derived from fats); intracellular messengers; insulation (e.g., fats prevent body heat loss); and vitamin delivery (fat-soluble vitamins such as A, D, E, and K are carried by fats through the bloodstream). Triglycerides are the large portion of fats in fat tissues and in muscle tissues.

Almost all fats which are required for bodily functions can be synthesized in the body, with linoleic acid being the only possible exception. Therefore, the concept of essential versus non-essential fats is not as well defined as for amino acids. However as mentioned earlier, fat intake is needed for the absorption of fat-soluble vitamins. Fats are derived from meat, fish, poultry, and dairy products (e.g., butter).

Fats represent by far the largest source of stored energy in the body. In moderate exercise, energy is equally derived from carbohydrates and fats. During longer exercises (> 1 hr), carbohydrate resources are depleted, and fat utilization increases to up to 80% of all energy required. Endurance athletes can utilize more fats at an earlier stage of exercise, and thus can save carbohydrates for later use. The use of caffeine also increases early use of fats as a source of energy.

In intense exercise, energy is derived solely from carbohydrates. Carbohydrates are the only source of fuel that can be quickly mobilized for intense bouts of activities.

WATER AND ELECTROLYTES

Figure 8.2 summarizes the use of foodstuffs as a source of energy under aerobic and anaerobic conditions. Furthermore, the figure shows that exercise causes adaptation in the utilization of different amounts of the three sources of nutrition. Drugs and hormones similarly influence the ratio of utilization of these three sources of energy.

FOOD SUPPLEMENTS

Modern day literature has found that certain food supplements for athletes may contribute to optimal performance, especially for elite athletes. However, genetic predisposition, training, and mental preparation for the event play the largest role in optimal performance outcome. Moderate intake of car-

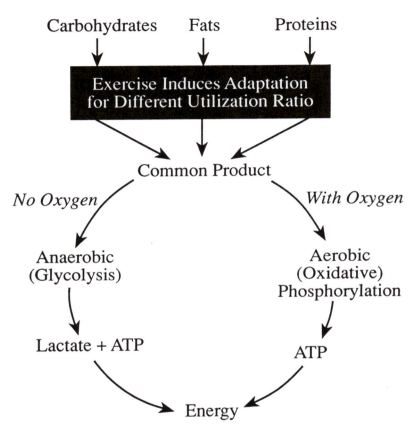

Figure 8.2. Flowchart of the metabolic pathways for foodstuff to energy production.

bohydrates as we maintained earlier is beneficial during the event. Also, moderate amounts of vitamins (one a day multivitamins for insurance) and antioxidants such as vitamin E and C (part of the multivitamins), beta-carotene, and selenium would be useful. The use of antioxidants is especially worthwhile since free radical damage to tissues is considered one of the causes of aging. Antioxidants are scavengers of free radicals. There is a great deal of quackery and hype regarding sports food supplements. Over nutrition of mega amounts could pose health risks to the athlete. Moderation is the message.

To date, much has been learned about the beneficial effects of calcium in the diet of young and old to help in bone formation and prevent bone loss with aging (i.e., osteoporosis). Nutritional guidelines released by the National Research Council in the summer of 1997 recommend that older women and men take in a total of 1,200 mg of calcium a day in the food that they eat or via a calcium supplement.

FURTHER GENERAL READING

Haymes, E.M. (1991) Vitamin and Mineral Supplementation to Athletes. Inter. J. Sports Nutrition 1(2):146–169.

Katch, F.I. and W.D. McArdle. (1993) Introduction to Nutrition, Exercise, and Health. 4th Edition, Lea and Febiger, Philadelphia, pp. 149–168.

Lemon, P.W.R. (1991) Protein and Amino Acid Needs of the Strength Athlete. Inter. J. of Sports Nutrition 1(2):127–145.

O'Neil F. et. al. (1986). Research and Applications of Current Topics in Sports Nutrition. J. of the Am. Dietetic Assoc. 86:1007–1015.

Wolinsky, I. and Hickson, Jr., J.F., Editors, (1994). "Nutrition in Exercise and Sport," 2nd edition, CRC Press, Boca Raton, Florida, pp. 1–416.

Chapter

NINE

Gender Differences in Exercise and Aging

In the popular culture of America, and sometimes in the sporting world, women have been typically viewed "as the weaker sex/gender". However, regarding issues of aging, longevity, and the responses to exercise and training, this is not accurate. Women have a tendency to live significantly longer than men and have better immune systems. Furthermore, women have exactly the same capacity to adapt to aerobic and strength training programs as men and benefit from all forms of physical activity.

It is well-known that the aging rate is different in women and men. Usually the aging rate is measured as changes in the various physiological systems with time. Men age fairly consistently with time while women age more slowly between the ages of 45 and 60 years, and faster between the ages of 70 and 80 years. The experts in the area of population statistics tell us that there are more males born than females, but there are more male stillbirths and miscarriages. Females not only have a "survival advantage" at birth, but throughout life and aging. On a worldwide basis, women outlive men by an average of 4 to 10 years. Therefore, it appears that maybe men are the weaker gender in our species. The reasons given for why women live significantly longer than men include genetic differences in the Y chromosome that only men have, hormonal differences, and the fact that women generally lead less stressful lives than do men. Also, until fairly recently, there were many more male smokers than female, and males had significantly greater rates of heart disease. Now that more women smoke, the experts see the rates of heart disease becoming much more similar in women and men. What is interesting is that if you look at the average length of life over 6 decades in the U.S., it directly mirrors the smoking trends in the general population. One could therefore say that there are definite gender differences in survival and longevity but that smoking is a lifestyle habit does not discriminate; it is the great equalizer between the sexes as a cause of death.

There are other interesting healthcare-related facts about men and women and aging. Older women usually have more contact with the health care system than men and more acute illnesses. Women are also more likely to have arthritis, sinus infections, colon inflammation, soft tissue disorders, and chronic constipation. That's the bad news, for the supposedly weaker sex. The good news is that while they do have a tendency to get sick more frequently, women generally have better and faster immune systems. On the macho side, men still have greater rates of emphysema and cardiovascular problems like heart disease and hypertension. Women usually lose height faster than men due to osteoporosis (bone loss) and the accompanying compression fractures of the spine. As far as body composition is concerned, at the age of 70 years, women on average have about 39% fat where men are only 21% fat. In men with aging, there is an increase in fat accumulation around the waist and mid section, and internally around the organs with a decrease in fat under the surface of the skin on the arms and legs. In women, the fat under the surface of the skin stays fairly constant after 45 years of age but the increase in total body fat is due to an increase in internal fat around the organs. It should be mentioned at this point that the fat you can see around the waist and under the surface of the skin is not as detrimental to health status as the internal fat around the organs that contributes to abnormal fat metabolism and problems with levels of fats and cholesterol in the blood.

One question that has been answered only quite recently is whether older men and women show similar improvements in physical fitness after aerobic and strength training. When older women and men perform regular, moderately intense aerobic exercise training for 10–12 weeks they both have about a 15–20% increase in cardiovascular fitness as measured by their maximal oxygen consumption. The interesting thing about this basic fact is that the amount of improvement is not only the same for older women and men but similar to the improvements seen in young sedentary individuals in their 20's and 30's. Generally speaking, men are physically stronger than women at both young ages and in older folks as well. Part of this difference in strength has to do with body size, plus the fact that in our society men, more often than women, perform physical activities requiring strength. Also, hormonal factors like the level of testosterone in the blood of men stimulate muscles to get bigger. When older men and women perform moderate strength training over the period of 2–3 months, there is about a 20–40% increase in muscle strength in both sexes. So as you can see, even though men are stronger than women, improvements are similar. There is even some research to show that women improve more in strength after exercise training because they are not as strong to begin with. The other aspect about gender differences with regard to strength is that even with very strenuous weight training that shows big gains in muscle strength, women very seldom develop large muscles (i.e., hypertrophy), again due to hormonal differences between the sexes. Are women really the "weaker" gender? They are usually smaller in stature and less strong **BUT**, they live longer and improve their fitness levels and benefit from regular exercise training programs just as much as men do.

FURTHER GENERAL READING

Spirduso, W.W. (1995) Individual Differences, Chapter 2, In: Physical Dimensions of Aging, Human Kinetics, Champaign, IL, pp. 33–56.

Spirduso, W.W. (1995) The Physically Elite Elderly, Chapter 14, In: Physical Dimensions of Aging, Human Kinetics, Champaign, IL, pp. 389–417.

Wells, C.L. (1991) Women, Sport, and Performance: A Physiological Perspective (2nd Edition), Human Kinetics, Champaign, IL.

Chapter

TEN

Diseases Associated with the Aging Process and the Effects of Exercise Training

A number of the diseases that affect the population by decreasing general health, lessening productivity, adding to the health care cost burden of the nation, and impacting the quality of life of individuals are associated with the aging process. Coronary artery disease, high blood pressure, diabetes, obesity, and osteoporosis all fit into this category, and were once thought to be inevitable consequences of the aging process. In studying many healthy older individuals and older master athletes who have maintained optimal eating habits, a relatively stable body weight through the years and performed regular, moderate aerobic and strength training exercise, we now know that in many cases the severity of these diseases can be reduced in many people. For some individuals, optimal lifestyle habits performed over the lifetime may be so powerful as to prevent the occurrence of these diseases completely.

There are a number of diseases that are thought by many in the medical profession to be conditions that normally occur with aging. Diseases such as coronary artery disease, hypertension, type II or adult-onset diabetes, osteoporosis, sarcopenia or muscle wasting, obesity, and arthritis are often viewed as natural processes that most people suffer with as they get older. However, there are older people who for either genetic or lifestyle reasons bypass these debilitating conditions that limit one's physical capacity and interfere with the older person's quality of life. One group of older adults seems to have less coronary artery disease, lower blood pressure, better sugar metabolism and bone density, more optimal body fat levels, and better muscular function than aged-matched subjects of the same gender. These older adults are called master athletes by most of the scientists who study them since they are usually between the ages of 40 and 80 years old. These master athletes are folks who either have performed regular sports training since their formative years or people who have taken up exercise training in their later years. Most often the master athletes are involved with distance running, cycling, swimming, triathlon competition, weight training, and cross country skiing to such an extent that they train very intensely on a daily basis and enter age group competitions on the local and national level. It is interesting to note that not only do these master athletes have lower incidences of the aforementioned diseases that we normally associate with aging than their age-matched but sedentary counterparts, but in many cases their health status is quite similar to young individuals who perform the same type and amount of exercise training. Thus it appears that regular exercise training does have the effect of improving overall health status in older people. Well then, what exactly are these age-related diseases and how does exercise help prevent or reduce their occurrence?

CORONARY ARTERY DISEASE

Coronary artery disease is a condition that causes a thickening of the blood vessel wall and the buildup of fatty blockages in the medium and large arteries that carry blood to the heart. When blood flow and oxygen delivery to the heart muscle is significantly reduced, the individual usually experiences chest pain, especially during exercise or while doing physical work. In situations where blood flow is completely blocked the individual may suffer a heart attack where areas of the heart muscle tissue actually dies. The blockages in the arteries are largely made up of cholesterol, a waxy substance that is carried in the blood by a protein molecule called LDL-cholesterol (low density lipoprotein, the so-called "bad cholesterol"). It is largely the LDL-cholesterol molecule that deposits cholesterol in the arteries.

Risk factors are characteristics that are directly related to the occurrence of a particular disease. The major risk factors for coronary artery disease are high blood pressure (hypertension), elevated blood cholesterol levels, smoking, and physical inactivity. Exercise training, especially aerobic exercise like running, walking, and cycling, has a beneficial effect on 2 of the major risk factors for coronary artery disease. First, exercise training can lower blood pressure in those individuals who have mild to moderate elevations at rest. More specifics on this in the next section. Secondly, aerobic exercise training can have a positive impact in cholesterol and fat levels in the blood. The scientific literature has shown that exercise training has little effect on the total amount of cholesterol or the amount of LDL-cholesterol in the blood of those who perform regular exercise. However, HDL-cholesterol levels do increase significantly with training. HDL-cholesterol (the "good" cholesterol) levels are important since it is the HDL molecule that picks up the cholesterol in the blood and carries it to the liver where it can be degraded and excreted from the body. Several studies have shown that about 10 miles per week of jogging or the equivalent in other modes of exercise are enough to significantly raise HDL-cholesterol levels in the blood. Another point is that the master athletes that we spoke of earlier tend to have cholesterol levels very similar to young sedentary subjects and aerobically trained athletes. Aerobic exercise training also reduces the triglyceride level (level of blood fat) significantly by about 20–30% in those who have elevated blood levels.

HYPERTENSION

High blood pressure is a major risk factor for heart disease and stroke and is currently a major public health problem in the U.S., with approximately 58 million people (that's 58,000,000) experiencing blood pressures that are elevated. Elevations in blood pressure are bad for older individuals because the increased pressure in the blood vessels increases the risk for stroke and coronary artery disease, as mentioned above. Two numbers are used to represent the pressure of the blood in the arteries, systolic pressure (which is the pressure in the vessels when the heart muscle is contracting) and diastolic pressure (which is measured when the heart is relaxing). The upper limits of normal blood pressure measured in millimeters of mercury (mmHg) are systolic blood pressure of 140 over a diastolic pressure of 90 (i.e., 140/90 mmHg). In many people, at rest the values can reach to 160–180 over 90–110 mmHg, levels that most cardiologists would not let their patients exercise with until the pressures were reduced. Generally, the safe cutoff for allowing people to exercise is below 160/95. Regular aerobic exercise training, weight loss in the vicinity of 20 lbs. or so, and salt restricted diets can lower blood pressure in humans by about 10 mmHg. Medicine is prescribed for those individuals who have a more severely elevated case of high blood pressure or for those who don't respond to the exercise/weight loss/low salt diet course of treatment.

DIABETES

Diabetes is a disease characterized by elevated blood sugar levels and either very high or very low insulin levels. When the elevated blood sugar occurs in children it is usually due to the lack of insulin production by the pancreas. This is referred to as juvenile-onset or Type I diabetes with the treatment usually consisting of regular injections of the hormone insulin that helps glucose/sugar to be taken up into muscle and fat cells. However, 85% of the people afflicted with diabetes have Type II, or adult-onset diabetes, where blood levels of glucose are elevated because the tissues are insensitive to the insulin that is present in the blood. It is Type II diabetes that is the problem for older individuals. The elevated glucose and insulin levels result in damage to the very small capillaries that carry blood to various tissues including the eye, kidney, heart, fingers, and toes, where nerves can also be injured. Thus, if gone undiscovered for a long time, diabetes can result in blindness, kidney disease, and the loss of limbs due to death of tissue, i.e., amputation of toes/feet and the entire lower limb.

The cause of Type II diabetes is not completely known, but it is thought to be due to both genetic and environmental factors. The risk of developing diabetes is related to the duration, degree, and distribution of obesity with those individuals with excess fat in the abdominal region being more likely to contract the disease. In this context, fully 80% of patients with diabetes are obese, which results in elevated blood insulin levels at rest and tissue insensitivity to insulin.

One question to be answered is: Does physical activity or exercise training prevent or cure diabetes? Noted physician and physical activity/disease specialist Dr. Ralph Paffenbarger studied a larger number of male alumni from the University of Pennsylvania from 1962 to 1976 by giving the subjects physical activity questionaires and watching for the development of diabetes. Over this 14 year time span the researchers found that as the physical activity of the subjects increased (as measured by calories expended per week) the incidence or number of folks to develop diabetes decreased. Thus, physical activity was thought to have a protective effect against the development of diabetes; this was especially true for those subjects who were obese. In 1991, the Nurses Health Study also showed that vigorous physical activity in 34–60 year old women reduced the risk of becoming diabetic over 8 years. These 2 studies taken together suggest that regular physical activity can reduce the risk of acquiring diabetes. Well then, what about the effects of exercise training in those who have already contracted the disease? Aerobic, and in some cases strength training have been shown to decrease the elevated insulin and glucose levels in the blood of persons with mild to moderate forms of diabetes. The effect is brought about by the fact that exercise increases the uptake of glucose into the tissues and increases the sensitivity of the tissues to insulin. The improvement in glucose metabolism for diabetics is even more pronounced when the physical activity program also brings about a loss of body fat. There are a couple of studies that show that very vigorous exercise can "cure" diabetes in those mildly afflicted but that once the exercise training is stopped, the elevated blood glucose levels return immediately.

OSTEOPOROSIS

Osteoporosis is a disease characterized by low bone density and a deterioration of bone leading to increased bone fragility and risk of fracture. It appears that post-menopausal women are at the greatest risk for developing osteoporosis and the most important factor that determines the risk for osteoporosis is the amount of bone mass that the individual has when they go through menopause. In terms of bone health it is imperative to attempt to maintain bone density or increase it in women between the ages of 35 and 50 years in those areas most susceptible to fracture, the lower lumbar spine, neck of the femur (upper leg bone), and the wrist. The few studies that have been done have shown that active women who perform regular physical exercise have greater bone density than sedentary women, and that sedentary women who perform exercise training show small but significant increases in bone density. One important point to emphasize here is that bone health is enhanced by weight bearing exercise, that is exercise against gravity or that exerts mechanical forces on the bone. Inactivity, immobilization, or extended periods of bed rest all result in decreases in bone mass.

   Many of the studies in young and older women have failed to show large increases in bone mineral density because either the type or length of training was insufficient or due to other factors, such as hormonal status and calcium intake. Activities like jogging, walking, stair climbing, and weight training are the most likely to elicit increases in bone density, but the activities probably have to be performed fairly vigorously and for a prolonged period of time in order to see results. In addition, the ability to increase bone mass may also be enhanced by taking supplemental calcium (~ 800–1,000 mg/day) and, if postmenopausal, going on hormone replacement therapy. Thus, in older women the optimal bone health program would include weight bearing exercise performed on a moderate level, calcium, and hormone treatment. Generally speaking, low bone density is not as much of a problem in older men as in women until men reach the age of 70 or so. In fact, several studies have shown that master athlete runners in their 60's have similar bone density as runners in their 20–30's who train the same amount. Whereas, young women in their 30–40's would be well advised to start following an optimal bone health program prior to reaching menopause, older men may not **have** to follow such a regimen until a later time. Having said that, it is probably also true that it would be more effective for men to perform regular exercise training for bone maintenance and other reasons, as mentioned previously, rather than try to increase bone density to a large degree later in life.

OBESITY

Obesity, defined as an excess of adipose or fat tissue, is another major public health problem in the United States that plays a major role in the development of diabetes, and increases the risk for coronary heart disease, high blood pressure, osteoarthritis, abnormal blood lipids, and certain forms of cancer. Progressive weight gain in the form of fat occurs between age 30 and 60 primarily due to decreases in physical activity which is somewhat amazing since energy intake also declines over this period of time. This means that the amount of exercise must decrease more than the calories taken in. According to the recent Surgeon General's Report on Physical Activity and Health (1996), in 1991 about 33% of adults in this country were overweight, this translates into about 60 million people who weigh too much. Furthermore, from 1976 to 1991 the average weight of American adults increased by over 8 pounds. An increase in body fat occurs when energy intake in the form of calories eaten exceeds the daily energy output over a prolonged period of time.

Energy output or expenditure is the total number of calories expended per day and is made up of calories "burned" while at rest, extra calories burned as a result of eating when the metabolic rate is increased about 10%, and the calories expended as a result of physical activity. This energy balance equation looks like this:

Calories In = *Calories Out* ☞ **No change in body weight**

But if:

Calories In > *Calories Out* ☞ **Increase in body weight**

Also:

Calories In < *Calories Out* ☞ **Decrease in body weight**

Obviously, above equations number 1 and 3 are the optimal situation in the real world and since so many older adult individuals are overweight, people should zero in on equation number 3. One basic fact to know concerning weight loss is that 1 pound of fat energy is stored for every 3,500 calories of excess energy intake. Also, 3,500 calories of energy must be expended via exercise training or physical activity to lose one pound of fat. As far as activity goes, it would take 35 miles of running or jogging to expend 3,500 calories or 100 miles of cycling at 10 MPH.

Many studies over the last 20 years have been carried out to determine the effects of exercise training on body weight and obesity, most of the studies were in young to middle-aged individuals but more recently, older people have been studied. The bottom line is that physical activity promotes fat loss while maintaining lean muscle tissue; weight loss is directly related to the frequency and duration of the training sessions and to the duration of training in months and years of the program. The combination of increases in physical activity and dieting is the most effective for long term weight regulation. It should be pointed out here that in terms of weight loss, all forms of exercise training are not created equal. For best results in a weight loss program, it is best to focus on aerobic forms of exercise training like walking/jogging/cycling, etc. since relatively few- calories are expended in strength training unless the participant is training many hours a day.

FURTHER GENERAL READING

Leon, A.S. (1997) Physical Activity and Cardiovascular Health: A National Consensus, Human Kinetics, Champaign, IL., pp. 1–296.

McArdle, W.D., F.I. Katch, and V.L. Katch. (1996) Physical Activity, Health, and Aging. In: Exercise Physiology, 4th Edition, Williams and Wilkins, Baltimre, Chapter 30, pp. 646–653.

Wilmore, J.H. and D.L. Costill. (1994) Physical Activity for Health and Fitness. In: Physiology of Sport and Exercise, Human Kinetics Publishers, Champaign, IL. Section G, pp.-

GLOSSARY

acclimatization: the physiological process by which an organism "gets used to being" in the heat or in the cold so that the climate doesn't significantly affect them.

activities of daily living (ADL): the life skills that everyone performs on a daily basis like eating, dressing, cleaning, shopping for food and other household tasks.

adipose: tissue composed of fat cells that store triglycerides.

aerobic: metabolism that utilizes oxygen to produce ATP for cellular or muscle work.

alveoli: small air sacs in the lungs where oxygen and carbon dioxide are exchanged with the blood.

American College of Sports Medicine (ACSM): the premier sports medicine organization in the world that is responsible for providing up to the minute information on exercise, training, nutrition and sports medicine related issues (www.ACSM.org).

amino acids: small organic compounds that are the building blocks for proteins. There are 20 amino acids.

anaerobic (exercise or metabolism): cellular processes occurring in the absence of oxygen. For example, in sprinting the muscles need for ATP is greater than the delivery system can provide sufficient oxygen. Thus carbohydrates are degraded without oxygen resulting in the formation of lactic acid (lactate).

analgesic: relieving pain (i.e. with the use of a drug).

anterior cruciate ligament: ligament that attaches the lateral side of the femur to the frontal side of the tibia.

anti-inflammatory: a medicine or treatment agent that reduces the degree of tissue inflammation.

ATP (Adenosine Triphosphate): An organic molecule used as the most prevalent energy currency in all cells of the body. It contains three phosphates linked together. The breakdown of the terminal phosphate releases energy utilized in numerous cellular functions. ATP is the source of energy for muscles.

autonomic nervous system: part of the nervous system that regulates involuntary body functions such as skeletal and cardiac muscles, smooth muscle (intestine) and glands. The system consists of two parts — the sympathetic nervous system in charge of increased heart rate, vasoconstriction and rise in blood pressure and the parasympathetic nervous system in charge of slowing down heart rate, increases intestinal movement, and increases gland function.

balance: a skill component of physical fitness having to do with the maintenance of a steady posture during standing or moving activity.

blood pressure: the hydrostatic pressure exerted by circulating blood against the walls of arteries.

blood volume: the volume of the entire blood in the body — about 5 liters for a 70 kg person.

body composition: a component of physical fitness that describes the relative proportions of fat, muscle, and bone of the body.

Bone: a lightweight structural scaffolding material which functions to support the body's tissues. It also acts as an anchoring point for muscles and ligaments. It has a high calcium content and functions as a reservoir for this mineral throughout the body. The end portions of bones which are associated with joints are coated with a relatively soft, smooth, low friction articular cartilage which may be damaged by injury or arthritis. Throughout the normal aging process, calcium and thus structural strength are gradually decreased within the bones. This is known as osteoporosis and occurs at a greater rate in women, especially those who are post menopausal.

bone density: the thickness of the bone tissue and amount of mineral content that gives structure to the bone.

bone scan: the use of a radioactive substance injected into the vein along with an imaging device in order to visualize bone structure and possible pathology.

bursa: small thin sac-like structures located in various areas throughout the body. They are present over surfaces which are prominent and subject to a significant amount of motion. Bursas are present over the prominence of the elbow, within the shoulder and over the front of the knee. When not injured, these structures are not noticed but when traumatized, they can become thickened, prominent and filled with fluid.

bursitis: bursitis develops from either an acute or chronic injury. The region of the affected bursa becomes inflamed and this is usually associated with a fluid build-up within the bursal sac noticed as swelling.

caffeine: a chemical compound found in coffee and chocolate. Caffeine is a central nervous system stimulant.

capillaries: small vessels that connect arteries and veins in tissues and muscles and allow the exchange of nutrients (e.g., oxygen, sugar) with waste products due to muscle activities.

carbohydrates: varied organic compounds such as saccharides and starches which serve as the main source of energy for the body. Gum and cellulose are also carbohydrates but humans lack the enzymes needed to digest them.

cardiac output: amount of blood pumped by the heart in liters/minute.

cardiovascular system: pertains to the heart and blood vessels. The heart pumps blood into vessels to deliver nutrients to muscles and tissues and removes waste products.

cartilage: There are two main types of cartilage present within the body. Articular or hyaline cartilage, as mentioned above lines the joint. Fibrocartilage is the other variety which is present in such areas as the intervertebral discs and the meniscus in the knee. Those structures function as shock absorbers and stabilizers within the knee, back, etc. Cartilage in general has a very limited capacity for self-repair, and therefore, in many instances, will require surgical treatment, when injured.

collagen: the major protein of connective tissue.

compartment syndrome: an increased compression of the artery resulting in reduced blood flow. This is a serious pathology that could cause permanent damage to the hand or foot.

contusion: Any blunt injury or blow to an area of the body will cause a contusion. This will lead to injuries of the subcutaneous tissue, muscle and possible nearby tendons. Recent

MRI studies have also shown that even bones can sustain contusions or bruises. Surrounding bleeding occurs as well as swelling, pain and discoloration. Usually these injuries will resolve with appropriate rest, ice, elevation, etc.

coronary artery disease: blockages made up of cholesterol deposits in the large arteries that serve the heart.

cryo-therapy: the use of cold temperature (i.e., ice) to lower metabolism in therapy of muscle injury.

dehydration: loss of water from the watery portion of the blood and cells, serious medical problem.

deltoid ligament: the medial ligament of the ankle joining medial malleolus with talus.

detraining: changes in the body's structure or function that occurs when regular physical training ceases or is reduced.

diabetes: abnormal glucose/sugar metabolism that results in very high blood sugar levels and either very low or very high insulin levels. Type II diabetes is the form of the disease that is usually acquired with aging.

diastolic: blood pressure in the arteries when the heart is not contracting.

digitalis: a drug made from the foxglove plant that strengthens heart muscle contractions that is usually given in emergency situations and to heart patients.

dislocations: Dislocations usually occur due to significant trauma. They are present when one or more bones are displaced out of their appropriate joints. They most commonly occur within the shoulder, but can occur in almost any location in the body. The bones may or may not spontaneously return to the normal position. Nonetheless, the surrounding ligaments and tissues are usually significantly damaged at the time of injury and require treatment. Occasionally, muscle relaxants, anesthesia and knolwedgeable traction and manipulation are required to reduce joints. When a dislocation is incomplete and the bone only comes part way out of the joint, this is termed a subluxation and can be more difficult to diagnose.

duration: the length of time of an exercise session, usually in minutes.

EKG: electrocardiography, the measurement of the electrical activity of the heart.

elasticity: the quality of muscle that allows it to yield to passive physical stretching.

electrolytes: salts in solutions (i.e. body fluid) which dissociate into ions. For example, in such solution table salt dissociates into sodium ions (Na^+) and chloride ions (Cl^-). Body fluid electrolytes include Na^+, Cl^-, K+, Mg^{2+}, Ca^{2+} and others. The maintenance of certain concentrations of electrolytes inside versus outside the cell is critical in maintaining the viability and function of the cell.

endorphin: chemical compounds (neuro peptides) secreted in the brain. endorphins have many effects on the body; among them, feeling high, and analgesia. endorphins are released during exercise.

endurance: ability of a person to perform a prolonged sporting event without adverse effects such as fatigue, exhaustion, or injury.

energy expenditure: the amount of energy consumed while at rest or during activity. The unit of energy is the kilocalorie (kcal) which is = to 1 Calorie = 4.184 kilojoules.

enzyme: a protein that catalyzes (speeds up) a chemical reaction in various metabolic pathways. In exercise physiology the pathways and enzymes of glycolysis and oxidative phosphorylation are the most important.

ergogenic aids: any substance or treatment that enhances the ability to achieve a greater work output.

ergometer: an athletic device or machine that has the ability to measure work output, as in a bicycle ergometer or a rowing/skiing ergometer etc.

exercise: a planned, structured bout of physical activity performed to improve physical fitness.

exercise prescription: an organized, individualized plan for exercise that describes the frequency, intensity, duration, and progression of an exercise session and a training program.

exercise training: bouts of physical activity that are performed repeatedly over time to improve or maintain physical fitness.

exercise-induced asthma: a constriction of air passages in the tracheal bronchial tree of the lungs experienced during exercise. Symptoms include: breathlessness, coughing and wheezing.

exercise physiologist: a professionally trained expert in the physiology of exercise and sports training.

fat: a substance made up of lipids and fatty acids. Certain fats are used as structural components of cells and as energy sources for metabolism.

flexibility: the "stretchiness" or ease of movement of a muscle or a joint. A flexible individual has a large range of motion at a joint.

Fractures: When bones are subject to a force greater than their strength, they will break. This is known as a fracture. Fractures can be simple, in which the skin and surrounding tissues are not violated, or they can be compound or open, in which a bone is protruding through the skin or exposed to the outside elements. Compound fractures are quite severe and require immediate operative care. Fractures can also be divided into displaced or non-displaced. Those fractures in which the bones are still well aligned may be treated with simple immobilization in a cast or brace until healing occurs. Those fractures which are displaced or angulated often require manipulation or surgical intervention to reposition and stabilize this position with plates, screws, rods, etc. A unique type of fracture is that of a stress fracture which is a localized failure of the bone due to repetitive over use trauma as occurs in running or excessive jumping. This type of fracture may or may not be visible on a routine x-ray and sometimes requires further studies. Stress fractures are common in the legs and feet. Rest or immobilization is required for healing.

frequency: the component of an exercise prescription that describes the number of times a person exercises, usually per week.

gerontologist: a practitioner or scientist who is an expert in the physiology, care and/or welfare of older individuals.

glucose: a simple sugar molecule found naturally in food such as fruits. It is a major source of energy in the muscle cell and the only source of energy for brain cells.

glycogen: a compound made from many glucose molecules strung together in a chain. It is the major form of stored energy in animal cells, especially in muscle and the liver.

glycogen loading: (or "super compensation") the process by which an athlete loads his muscle cells with extra glycogen by exercising vigorously several days before the day of the event and eating large amounts of carbohydrates followed by rest on the day before the event. This method stimulates the body to synthesize and store glycogen. In this manner, the athlete has a larger than normal amount of stored glycogen for utilization during the event.

glycolysis: a metabolic pathway involving the rapid breakdown of glucose to pyruvate without the presence of oxygen thus producing a rapid source of ATP for muscular work.

graded exercise test (GXT): An exercise test, usually performed on a motorized treadmill and supervised by a physician that is used to determine normal heart rate, blood pressure and EKG responses to increasing levels of exercise.

growth hormone (GH): a hormone secreted by the anterior pituitary portion of the brain that promotes bone and muscle tissue growth and protein synthesis.

heat cramps: a muscle spasm associated with pain due to excess heat that results in loss of water and reduced blood flow to the muscle.

heat exhaustion: caused by depletion of the body of water. Symptoms include weakness and malaise.

heat stroke: prolonged exposure to heat and sun resulting in dehydration and loss of the thermal regulatory function. Symptoms include a sense of impending doom, headache, dizziness, confusion, and weakness. It is a serious medical emergency that could cause death.

heart rate: frequency of heart muscle contraction (beats) per minute.

hematocrit: a measure of volume of packed cells in blood as percentage of blood volume. The normal range for men is 43%–49% and for women is 37%–43%.

hydrostatic pressure: amount of force exerted by a fluid (i.e., blood) per unit surface area of a vessel.

hyperinsulinemia: an excess amount of insulin secretion into the blood by the pancreas.

hyperlipidemia: high levels of fat in the blood, consisting of elevated triglycerides and lipoproteins.

hypertension: high blood pressure, usually considered to be blood pressure greater than 140/90 mmHg.

hypoglycemia: insufficient levels of sugar in the blood.

hypothalamus: a region in the brain involved in controlling body temperature, sleep, and appetite.

hypoxia: an insufficient concentration of oxygen in the tissue.

insulin: an important hormone secreted by the pancreas that stimulates glucose uptake into muscle and fat cells and facilitates glycogen storage.

intensity: the component of an exercise prescription that describes how hard a person is working, usually expressed as a % of maximal heart rate or VO_2 max for aerobic exercise training and as a % of 1 repetition maximum (RM) for resistive exercise.

ischemia: reduced blood flow to a tissue or organ, usually in reference to the heart (i.e. myocardial ischemia).

isokinetic: a muscular contraction that is performed at a constant velocity of limb movement.

isotonic: a muscle contraction that is performed against a constant external resistance.

isometric: a muscle contraction that generates force but cannot overcome the resistance thus resulting in no visible shortening of the muscle.

Krebs Cycle: a sequence of biochemical reactions that breakdown carbohydrates, fatty acids, and amino acids into carbon dioxide and water with the subsequent production of ATP (Adenosine Triphosphate = "the energy currency of the cell").

lactate (lactic acid): a metabolic molecule produced from the breakdown of glucose when muscles perform work in the absence of oxygen (an anaerobic process).

lactate threshold (LT): the work intensity that elicits significant lactate production that shows up and can be measured in the blood. LT usually occurs at between 60–80% of VO_2 max and can be increased with training.

ligament: Ligaments are fibrous structures similar to tendons. They, however, attach bones to one another as opposed to muscles to bones. Injuries to ligaments may often lead to instability or laxity of joints. Some ligaments have a capacity for healing on their own. Others may require definitive surgical treatment.

life span: the maximum number of years of life for a particular species.

lipoproteins: biochemical molecules that carry cholesterol in the blood.

longevity: the number of organisms living to old age in a species, i.e. the average age at death.

low back pain: usually chronic pain in the back that is due to excess weight carried in the front of the torso, weak abdominal muscles, sedentary occupations and poor posture while sitting.

luteinizing hormone (LH): a hormone secreted by the brain that stimulates the secretion of sex hormones in the ovary and testes.

magnetic resonance imaging (MRI): a non-radioactive imaging technology that is used to "take pictures" of the brain, muscles, joints, and internal organs for the purpose of locating pathologies.

master athlete: an individual who trains and competes on a regular basis in some form of athletic or physical activity.

maximal heart rate: the highest heart rate that is obtained during maximal exercise.

maximal oxygen consumption (VO_2 max): the organism's maximal capacity to take in, transport and utilize oxygen on the cellular level to generate ATP; the units of oxygen consumption are milliliters/kilogram/minute, i.e., ml/kg/min.

medial: toward the midline.

metabolism: refers to all biochemical processes in the body that are involved in areas such as growth, development, energy production, and repair.

MET: a unit of metabolism that is used to estimate the metabolic cost of an activity. 1 MET is the oxygen consumption at rest which is about 3.5ml O_2/kg/minute. 10 METS would correspond to an estimated metabolic cost of 35 ml O_2/kg/minute.

micro circulation: refers to the blood flow of smaller blood vessels such as capillaries. This system allows for the exchange of oxygen from blood to the tissues and the removal of waste products of exercise such as carbon dioxide and lactate from the tissue.

mitochondria: a small structure in the cell specializing in the production of ATP (Adenosine Triphosphate). i.e. "the power-house of the cell".

mode of exercise: the type of exercise, i.e., jogging, swimming or cycling etc.

motor unit: a motor nerve cell and the muscle fibers that are connected to it.

muscle: specialized elongated cells that have the capability to contract and relax, thus causing movement.

muscle fiber type (Type I, II): the percentage of Type I, slow twitch/oxygen utilizing fibers that are recruited during moderate intensity, prolonged bouts of exercise like cycling and distance running and swimming; and Type II or fast twitch cells that are recruited during activities like sprint running and swimming and intense weight lifting.

muscle size: the cross sectional area of a particular muscle.

muscle strength: the ability of a muscle to create tension or exert force against a resistance.

myelination: a sheath of tissue surrounding the nerves acting as an electrical insulator.

myoglobin: carrier of oxygen in muscle. A counterpart to hemoglobin as the oxygen carrier in the blood.

obesity: an abnormally high level of body fat where the percentage is greater than ~ 25% in men and 35% in women.

oblique: somewhere between horizontal and perpendicular.

ossification: the formation of bone (mostly calcium deposits called calcification).

osteoporosis: loss of bone density usually associated with older women especially in the lumbar spine, the femur, the upper leg bone and the wrist.

overload principle: a gradual increase in workload which results in greater endurance, power, and muscle size.

overtraining: attempting to do more physical work than can be tolerated by the body.

oxidation: the breakdown of chemicals involving oxygen (oxygen receives an electron from hydrogen). Usually this process occurs in the mitochondria, the power house of the cell.

pH: a scale that represents the acidity of solutions (i.e. a measure of hydrogen ion concentration). A pH value of 7.0 is neutral, above 7.0 is alkaline, and below 7.0 is acidic.

phosphocreatine or creatine phosphate: a small organic compound with high energy that can quickly form adenosine triphosphate (ATP) as a source of energy when needed without going through aerobic or anaerobic systems.

phosphorylation: the addition of phosphate onto a compound.

physical activity: movement of the body that is produced by the contraction of muscles and results in an increase in energy expenditure.

physical fitness: the capacity of the individual to respond to and successfully perform a bout of physical activity.

plantar fascia: fibrous tissue that supports the bottom of the foot.

plasma: the straw-colored fluid portion of the blood consisting of water, electrolytes, proteins, glucose, and others (i.e., the liquid portion of the blood).

posterior: view from the back, opposite to anterior.

post-menopausal: period that occurs after the permanent cessation of the menstrual cycle.

progression: a principle of training that increasing the work rate or workload results in an overload to the system and an adaptation.

protein: a large naturally occurring compound consisting of many amino acids. Proteins are involved in most cellular functions such as enzymes, structure, antibodies, …etc.

quadriceps (muscle): the four components of muscle at the front of the thigh — vastus medialis, vastus lateralis, vastus intermedius, and rectus femoris.

rating of perceived exertion (RPE): the subjective grading of how hard a person is working during exercise; usually on a 6 to 20, or 1 to 10 scale as devised by Dr. Gunnar AV Borg; also known as the Borg Scale. For most individuals a rating of 12–15 is optimal during a typical exercise training session.

repetition: the number of times a weight is lifted or an exercise is repeated.

repetition maximum: the maximal amount of weight that can be lifted a certain number of times, referred to as an RM; 1 RM is the maximal amount of weight that can be lifted one time. A 1 RM test is commonly used to measure muscle strength on several pieces of strength equipment or with free weights.

resistance: the force or weight against which a muscle must act in order to do work.

respiratory system: breathing system including the nose, mouth, trachea (windpipe), bronchi (tubes) and alveoli (air sacs of the lungs).

resting heart rate: the heart rate recorded when the person is completely at rest, usually between ~ 60–80 beats/minute.

risk factors: characteristics or behaviors that when present increase the probability of incurring some disease, e.g. a high blood cholesterol level is a *risk factor* for coronary artery disease.

sedentary: a person who performs no regular, meaningful physical activity.

serum: the remaining liquid after blood clots. When blood clots, it separate the solid components such as blood cells, platelets, and clotting factors from the remaining fluid called serum.

set: a unit of exercise consisting of a particular number of repetitions.

shin splint: tendonitis (inflammation) of the tibial or front area of the lower leg.

shock: collapse and sudden inability of the cardiovascular system to provide enough blood circulation to the body.

specificity principle: a training model that emphasizes that training must resemble the sporting activity for which the individual is training.

sprain: Sprains are injuries which occur to ligaments. They usually are the result of trauma and can be of varying degrees of severity. A grade I sprain is a mild stretch to a ligament, a grade II sprain is a more serious stretch injury which results in mild to moderate laxity (looseness) and a grade III sprain is a complete disruption of the ligament which may lead to a dis-location or gross instability. Ligament injuries may be treated with rest, therapy, and immobilization. Surgery may be required in certain anatomic areas.

starch: the main storage food in plants. It consist of long chains of glucose molecules. The counterpart to starch in animals is glycogen.

static stretching: stretching the muscle to a position of slight discomfort and holding it at that position for a period of time.

steroids: chemicals that share common structure with the steroid hormones.

steroid hormones: natural hormones in the body such as androgens and estrogens involved in sex characteristics and other important functions.

strain: Strains are injuries to the musculo-tendinous unit and result from an excessive force being applied to a muscle or tendon. These forces can result in an actual disruption or tear in the structure. If this occurs in the tendon or at its junction to bone, surgical repair may be required. Lesser injuries resulting in only a stretch to these structures, especially those within the muscle, often will heal with appropriate conservative measures.

stress fracture: microscopic cracks in a bone caused by excess-ive forces placed on the bone such as in prolonged running on hard pavement or repetitive jumping, often associated with dull aches and pains, usually in the bones of the foot and lower limb.

stroke volume: the amount of blood ejected per heart beat measured in milliliters.

sub-luxation: partial dislocation.

synovial (fluid): lubricating fluid in the joints.

systolic: pressure of the blood in the arterial vessels when the heart is contracting.

tendon: fibrous structures present throughout the body which serve to anchor the contractile muscles to bone. For example, the Achilles tendon anchors the calf muscles to the bone of the heel. Tendons can be injured or torn with acute traumatic injuries. Age-related breakdown can occur within the cellular structures of the tendons and eventually this may lead to a failure of the tendon and loss of its associated muscular function.

tendinitis: This is the condition which occurs when a tendon is irritated or inflamed. It can be caused either by a direct injury or chronic repetitive overuse injury. Tendinitis often causes localized swelling and pain.

thermo regulatory system: a structure located in the hypothalamus responsible for the regulation of normal body temperature.

triglycerides: Storage form of fat in muscle and fat cells, consisting of a fatty acid molecule and a compound called glycerol.

vasoconstriction: narrowing of the blood vessels that reduces blood flow.

vasodilation: increase in the diameter of the blood vessels that increases blood flow.

viscosity: thickness of a fluid that allows it to flow easily, as in the blood viscosity allowing for flow through the veins and capillaries. Blood that is too viscous or has a high viscosity doesn't flow well.

Index